Fluorescent Imaging: Treatment of Hepatobiliary and Pancreatic Diseases

Frontiers of Gastrointestinal Research

Vol. 31

Series Editor

Choitsu Sakamoto Tokyo

Fluorescent Imaging

Treatment of Hepatobiliary and Pancreatic Diseases

Volume Editors

Norihiro Kokudo Tokyo
Takeaki Ishizawa Tokyo

34 figures, 23 in color, and 8 tables, 2013

KARGER

Basel · Freiburg · Paris · London · New York · New Delhi · Bangkok · Beijing · Tokyo · Kuala Lumpur · Singapore · Sydney

Frontiers of Gastrointestinal Research

Prof. Norihiro Kokudo, MD, PhD
Professor and Chairman
Hepato-Biliary-Pancreatic Surgery Division
Artificial Organ and Transplantation Division
Department of Surgery, Graduate School of Medicine
The University of Tokyo
Tokyo 113-8655
Japan

Dr. Takeaki Ishizawa, MD, PhD
Assistant Professor
Hepato-Biliary-Pancreatic Surgery Division
Artificial Organ and Transplantation Division
Department of Surgery, Graduate School of Medicine
The University of Tokyo
Tokyo 113-8655
Japan

Library of Congress Cataloging-in-Publication Data

Fluorescent imaging: treatment of hepatobiliary and pancreatic diseases / volume editors, Norihiro Kokudo, Takeaki Ishizawa.
p. ; cm. -- (Frontiers of gastrointestinal research, ISSN 0302-0665 ; vol. 31)
Includes bibliographical references and indexes.
ISBN 978-3-318-02292-6 (hard cover : alk. paper) -- ISBN 978-3-318-02293-3 (electronic version)
I. Kokudo, Norihiro, editor of compilation. II. Ishizawa, Takeaki, editor of compilation. III. Series: Frontiers of gastrointestinal research ; v. 31. 0302-0665
[DNLM: 1. Biliary Tract Diseases--surgery. 2. Liver Diseases--surgery. 3. Digestive System Surgical Procedures--methods. 4. Optical Imaging--methods. 5. Pancreatic Diseases--surgery. W1 FR946E v.31 2013 / WI 770]
RD546
617.5'56--dc23
2013019195

Bibliographic Indices. This publication is listed in bibliographic services, including Current Contents® and Index Medicus.

www.karger.com
Printed in Germany on acid-free and non-aging paper (ISO 9706) by Kraft Druck, Ettlingen
ISSN 0302–0665
e-ISSN 1622–3754
ISBN 978–3–318–02292–6
e-ISBN 978–3–318–02293–3

Contents

Near-Future Technology

Preface

I do not recall the exact date, but I clearly remember how excited we were to find an 'illuminated' liver tumor in the OR one day in 2007. It was several weeks later that we started a prospective study on intraoperative ICG fluorescence cholangiography during liver surgery. We injected 100-fold diluted ICG solution via a tube inserted into the cystic duct to obtain anatomical information on the biliary tree. The patient had a recurrent hepatocellular carcinoma (HCC). Following cholecystectomy and insertion of a C-tube, we applied a near-infrared camera for fluorescence cholangiography. Immediately after the intrabiliary injection of ICG, we could identify the biliary tree, as expected. At the same time, however, we also found that the tumor itself was illuminating! Wait a second, has the tumor not been fluorescing from before the injection of ICG into the cystic duct? Instantly, we realized that the fluorescence of the tumor originated, in all likelihood, not from the ICG that we injected intraoperatively into the cystic duct, but from the ICG that we had injected 1 week before the operation as part of preoperative liver function testing.

It was then quite natural for liver surgeons to hypothesize that HCC cells can also take up ICG, just like hepatocytes, from which they arise. Normal hepatocytes quickly excrete ICG into the bile, so that they no longer illuminate fluorescence 1 week after the ICG injection. On the other hand, in the case of HCC cells, possibly on account of the disturbed excretory function of the cells, ICG excretion may be impaired and the ICG may be retained for weeks in the HCC cells. So far, evidence supports this aforementioned hypothesis, and molecular analyses on the genes encoding the transporters of this dye may help in a clearer elucidation of this phenomenon in the near future.

ICG is an old friend for hepatobiliary surgeons. It received FDA approval for clinical use more than half a century ago, and has been a very useful dye for liver function testing. ICG fluorescence angiography was applied first for visualizing the retinal artery by ophthalmologists in the late 1960s. It was then applied to the study of cerebral arteries, coronary arteries, limb arteries, mesenteric arteries, etc. With recent advances in imaging technologies, ICG has received renewed attention in the field of hepatobiliary surgery as a new tool for visualizing the biliary tree and liver tumors. What is unfortunate for this very useful dye in medicine, however, is that it is very cheap and is available for only JPY 644 (approximately USD 6.33 or EUR 4.89) for a 25-mg vial. The price is so low that no pharmaceutical company in the world has shown any interest in conducting expensive clinical trials to expand the clinical indications for the use of ICG.

This book on fluorescence imaging in the field of hepatobiliary and pancreatic diseases introduces cutting-edge knowledge about the exciting imaging technique using ICG and other new promising chemicals. I would like to thank all of the contributors for sharing their latest findings. I hope this book will encourage not only researchers, but also entrepreneurs, to promote technical developments and popularization of this technology. Lastly, I would like thank Dr. Takeaki Ishizawa, the co-editor of this book and a brilliant colleague of mine, as well as S. Karger Medical and Scientific Publishers for their energetic work in publishing this wonderful book.

Norihiro Kokudo, MD, PhD, Tokyo

Kokudo N, Ishizawa T (eds): Fluorescent Imaging: Treatment of Hepatobiliary and Pancreatic Diseases.
Front Gastrointest Res. Basel, Karger, 2013, vol 31, pp 1–9 (DOI: 10.1159/000348600)

History and Basic Technique of Fluorescence Imaging for Hepatobiliary-Pancreatic Surgery

Takeaki Ishizawa · Norihiro Kokudo

Hepato-Biliary-Pancreatic Surgery Division, Department of Surgery, Graduate School of Medicine, The University of Tokyo, Tokyo, Japan

Abstract

Recently, fluorescence imaging using indocyanine green (ICG) has been used clinically to visualize the vascular/lymphatic anatomy and cancerous tissues in real time during surgery. Potentially, among the best indications for ICG fluorescence imaging are hepatobiliary and pancreatic diseases since not only the fluorescent property of ICG but also its biliary excretion property can be utilized for imaging. In fact, ICG fluorescence imaging is already being used in clinical settings to identify the anatomy of the bile duct during laparoscopic surgery as well as open surgery in cases of liver cancer. 5-aminolevulinic acid is another fluorescent probe that has been administered to humans for identification of malignant glioma, bladder cancer and epidermal tumor, although its application to hepatobiliary and pancreatic diseases has rarely been evaluated. Preclinically, numerous kinds of novel fluorescent probes are being developed to improve the sensitivity and specificity of ICG fluorescence imaging, making in vivo fluorescence imaging one of the most active research fields in the world.

In vivo fluorescence imaging, aimed at delineating cancerous tissues and anatomic structures for accurate diagnosis and surgical treatment, has become one of the most active areas of medical research. Among the enormous amount of basic research being published, however, very few techniques have reached the level of clinical use, except for real-time fluorescence imaging techniques using indocyanine green (ICG) and 5-aminolevulinic acid (5-ALA). Herein, we review the history of research on fluorescence imaging techniques using ICG and 5-ALA, and introduce recent advances in the development of novel fluorescent probes that could be applied in the near future to the management of hepatobiliary and pancreatic diseases.

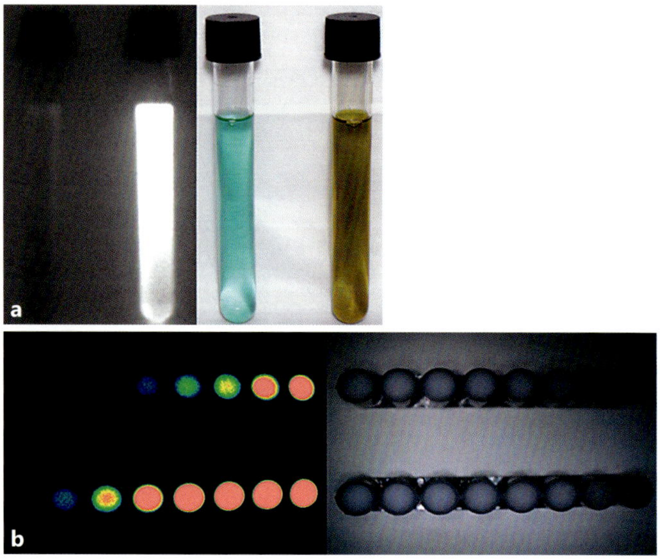

Fig. 1. In vitro fluorescence images of ICG solutions (left) and their gross appearance (right). **a** Although pure ICG solution (0.025 mg/ml) does not show fluorescence (left test tube), it begins to emit strong fluorescence following addition of a small amount of human bile (right test tube). **b** Increasing fluorescence intensity according to the ICG concentrations is visualized on pseudocolor images (left). In the present series, the highest fluorescence intensity was observed at the ICG concentration of 0.025 mg/ml.

Indocyanine Green

For more than 50 years since its approval by the Food and Drug Administration (FDA) in 1954, ICG has been used in clinical settings mainly to estimate cardiac output and liver function. The fluorescence property of ICG was characterized in detail in the 1970s, i.e. protein-bound ICG emits fluorescence that peaks at about 840 nm when illuminated with near-infrared light (750–810 nm; fig. 1) [1]. Because this wavelength is hardly affected due to absorption by hemoglobin or water, structures that contain ICG can be visualized through connective tissue thicknesses of up to 5–10 mm by combined use of an appropriate filter and a camera that is sensitive to the infrared region.

By utilizing the potential of ICG as a fluorescent probe to delineate biological structures, fluorescence imaging using ICG began to be applied clinically to fundus angiography in the field of ophthalmology in the early 1990s [2]. In the 21st century, the application of ICG fluorescence imaging has been extended to the field of surgery, as an intraoperative navigation tool to determine the lymphatic flow in the extremities [3], identify sentinel lymph nodes in patients with breast [4] and gastric cancer [5], and track blood flow during coronary artery bypass grafting [6] and clipping of cerebral artery aneurysms [7]. Little attention, however, has been paid to the fluorescence property of ICG in the fields of hepatobiliary and pancreatic surgery (probably because ICG has been widely adopted as a reagent for measuring liver function), except for the use of portal injection of ICG during surgery as a dye to delineate hepatic segments to be resected. In the last years, though, some researchers revisited the first known property of ICG, i.e. its biliary excretion, and developed the technique of intraoperative fluorescence cholangiography (table 1) [8–10].

Table 1. Clinical applications of ICG fluorescence imaging in hepatobiliary and pancreatic surgery

Reference	Indications	Concomitant use
Identification of hepatic segment		
Aoki et al. [35]	liver resection	
Uchiyama et al. [36]	liver resection	
Kasuya et al. [37]	liver resection	
Ishizawa T et al. [38]	laparoscopic liver resection	
Cholangiography		
Mitsuhashi et al. [9]	open cholecystectomy	angiography
Ishizawa et al. [39]	liver resection and open cholecystectomy	
Ishizawa et al. [15]	laparoscopic cholecystectomy	
Aoki et al. [40]	laparoscopic cholecystectomy	identification of hepatic segments
Tagaya et al. [41]	open/laparoscopic cholecystectomy	angiography
Sakaguchi et al. [42]	liver resection	bile leak test
Mizuno and Isaji [43]	liver transplantation (donor)	
Ishizawa et al. [16]	single incision laparoscopic cholecystectomy	
Hutteman et al. [44]	pancreatoduodenectomy	
Kaibori et al. [45]	liver resection	bile leak test
Kawaguchi et al. [46]	liver resection and transplantation	angiography
Sherwinter [17]	laparoscopic cholecystectomy	
Identification of liver cancer		
Ishizawa et al. [11]	liver resection (HCC and colorectal metastasis)	
Gotoh et al. [12]	liver resection (HCC)	
Ishizawa et al. [47]	laparoscopic liver resection (HCC)	
Yokoyama et al. [13]	liver resection (metastasis of pancreatic cancer)	
Ishizuka et al. [48]	liver resection (colorectal metastasis)	
Satou et al. [49]	resection of extrahepatic metastasis of HCC	
Morita et al. [50]	liver resection (HCC)	
Identification of cholecystic venous flow		
Kai et al. [51]	open cholecystectomy	
Identification of cholestatic hepatic segments		
Harada, et al. [52]	liver resection (liver cancer and bile duct cancer)	
Identification of lymphatic drainage		
Hutteman et al. [44]	pancreaticoduodenectomy	
Hirono et al. [53]	pancreaticoduodenectomy	
Angiography		
Kubota et al. [8]	liver transplantation	
Kaneko et al. [54]	laparoscopic cholescystectomy	
Evaluation of liver function in veno-occlusive regions		
Kawaguchi et al. [55]	liver resection and transplantation	

HCC = Hepatocellular carcinoma.

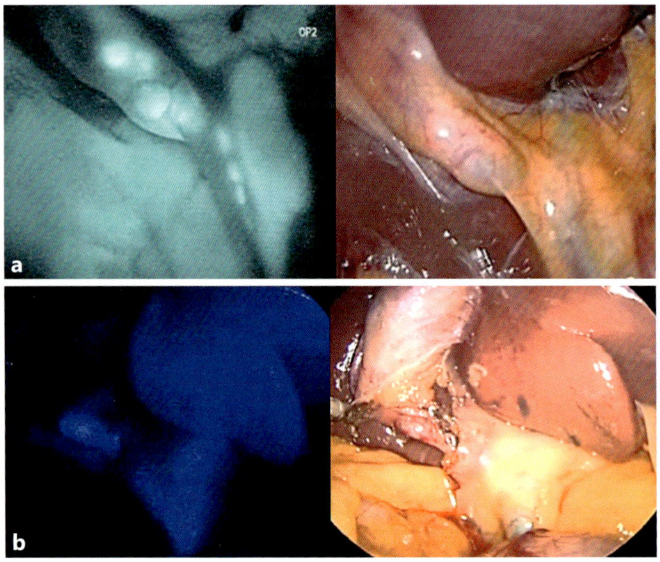

Fig. 2. Fluorescence cholangiography during laparoscopic cholecystectomy. **a** Fluorescence cholangiography before dissection of Calot's triangle using the 1-CCD fluorescence imaging system (Olympus Medical Systems, Tokyo, Japan). **b** Fluorescence cholangiography after dissection of Calot's triangle using the 3-CCD fluorescence imaging system (standard-definition model; Karl Storz, Tuttlingen, Germany).

As a navigational tool during surgery in patients with malignancy, the first clinical applications of ICG fluorescence imaging were identification of sentinel nodes in cases of breast and gastric cancer [4, 5]. Although intraoperative fluorescence imaging of lymph node distribution may have the potential to minimize the dissection area in surgeries for malignancies, fluorescence imaging does not reveal cancer-specific accumulation in metastatic lymph nodes – it only delineates the lymphatic drainage routes from the cancer tissue to the lymph nodes. By contrast, the nature of ICG fluorescence imaging of hepatocellular carcinoma, which was described for the first time in Japan in 2009 [11, 12], is very different from other fluorescence imaging techniques: it allows visualization of the hepatocellular carcinoma itself. Following intravenous administration, the ICG is taken up by the cancer cells, remaining in the cancer tissues at the time of surgery as a result of biliary excretion disorder.

Fluorescence imaging using preoperative intravenous administration of ICG also enables identification of small metastases in the liver, which are difficult to detect by visual inspection, palpation or ultrasonography during surgery [11, 13]. In the case of metastases, ICG accumulates not in the cancerous tissue itself, but in the noncancerous liver parenchyma surrounding the tumor, resulting in the appearance of rim fluorescence around the metastatic cancer on the cut surface of resected specimens [11].

Fluorescence imaging has the potential to be highly suitable for laparoscopic surgery, in which surgeons complete surgical procedures by video imaging. Indeed, since laparoscopic fluorescence imaging systems became commercially available in 2011, the ICG fluorescence imaging technique has begun to be applied to laparoscopic surgery in clinical settings not only in Japan [14–16], but also in the USA [17, 18], Switzerland [19] and Argentina [20], mainly as a tool for navigation of the bile duct anatomy during laparoscopic cholecystectomy (fig. 2). Another application of ICG fluorescence imaging is real-time microscopic visualization of the cellular structure during endoscopic or laparoscopic examinations, which may partly replace pathological diagnosis based on biopsy samples [21].

5-Aminolevulinic Acid

5-ALA is the natural precursor of the heme pathway. In noncancerous cells, exogenous application of 5-ALA results in production of protoporphyrin IX (PPIX) with a fluorescent property; however, PPIX is rapidly metabolized to nonfluorescent heme. In contrast, in malignant cells, administration of 5-ALA can cause overproduction of PPIX, probably as a result of increased activity of porphobilinogen deaminase and/or decreased activity of ferrochelatase [22, 23], enabling identification of cancerous tissues using 5-ALA-induced PPIX fluorescence.

Oral 5-ALA has been approved as an agent for photodynamic therapy of keratosis by the FDA and as an optical imaging agent for intraoperative identification of malignant glioma [24] in Europe and Korea. Intravesical administration of a 5-ALA derivative has also been used for the detection of bladder cancer [25]. However, there are few reports of fluorescence imaging using 5-ALA in the field of digestive surgery, except for its application to the detection of metastasis from gastric [26] and colorectal cancer [27]. A previous report revealed that the tissue concentration of protoporphyrin in the liver and pancreas gradually increases to reach its peak 7–10 h after oral administration of 5-ALA [28]. The author's group also confirmed fluorescence of PPIX in swine liver, pancreas and bile by naked-eye observation following oral 5-ALA administration (fig. 3), suggesting the potential use of 5-ALA as a fluorescent agent for intraoperative navigation during hepatobiliary and pancreatic surgery. The major advantage of 5-ALA-induced PPIX fluorescence is that it lies within optical regions (excitation: 440 nm; emission: 575–675 nm), while this fluorescent property may also pose a limitation with respect to tissue permeability to delineate deeply located cancerous tissues and bile ducts covered with connective tissue.

Novel Fluorescent Probes

Recently, there have been reports on numerous kinds of novel fluorescent probes for in vivo imaging of biological structures every month. Among these, close-to-clinical application techniques are introduced herein (please see the section 'Near-future technology').

One of the most promising indications of intraoperative fluorescence imaging is fluorescence cholangiography to avoid bile duct injury, or at least reduce the need for conventional radiological cholangiography during laparoscopic cholecystectomy, which has become one of the most popular surgical procedures worldwide. Although

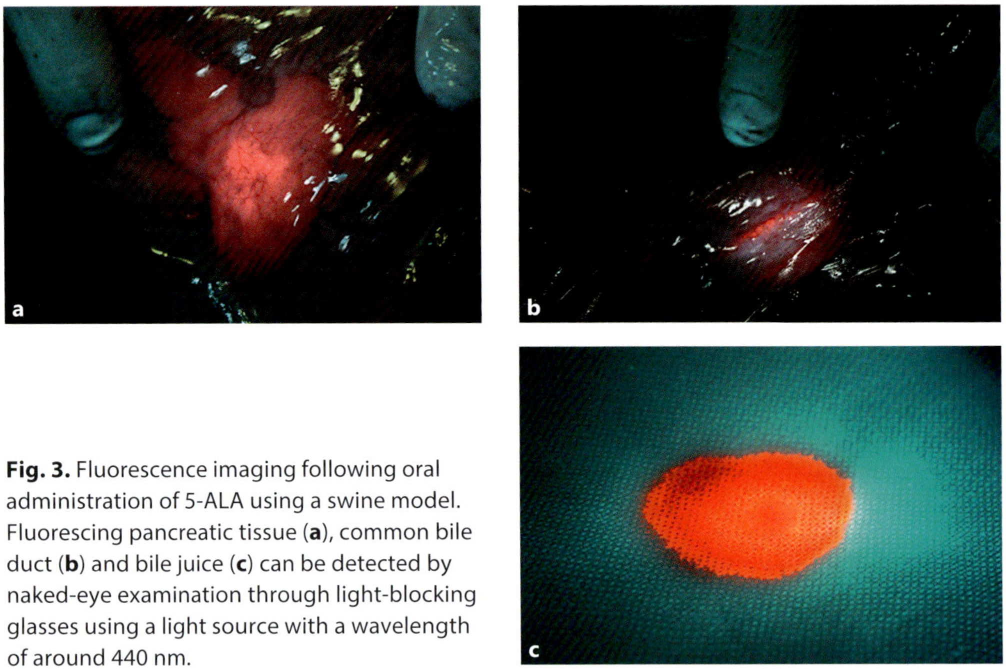

Fig. 3. Fluorescence imaging following oral administration of 5-ALA using a swine model. Fluorescing pancreatic tissue (**a**), common bile duct (**b**) and bile juice (**c**) can be detected by naked-eye examination through light-blocking glasses using a light source with a wavelength of around 440 nm.

ICG seems to have ideal properties for fluorescence cholangiography, novel preclinical agents with optimized pharmacokinetics and tissue permeability have also been developed for use in fluorescence cholangiography [29]. Frangioni and colleagues [30] have developed novel fluorescent probes to be used with ICG and/or methylene blue for simultaneous identification of the bile duct and vascular anatomy using a dual-channel near-infrared imaging system.

Considering the fact that ICG is almost the only fluorescent agent that can be administered intravenously to human subjects and will therefore remain the mainstay for the next few decades, Kobayashi and colleagues [31] at the National Institutes of Health continue to develop antibody-ICG conjugates to visualize specific receptor expressions in cancerous tissues in real time. In contrast, another group has produced novel fluorescent agents by conjugating known antigenic carbohydrates, such as carcinoembryonic antigen, with commercially available fluorophores other than ICG, enabling detection of metastatic lesions from pancreatic cancer in animal models [32]. Instead of utilizing the antigen-antibody reactions between fluorescent agents and cancerous tissues, Urano et al. [33] focused on cancer-specific overexpression of membrane enzymes and developed γ-glutamyl hydroxymethyl rhodamine green, which is completely quenched by spirocyclic caging, but is activated rapidly by a one-step enzymatic reaction in the presence of γ-glutamyltranspeptidase. This kind of probe may be applicable not only to detection of cancerous tissues overexpressing γ-glutamyltranspeptidase [34] during digestive surgery, but also for real-time visualization of pancreatic leaks based on the peptidase activities in pancreatic juice.

Conclusion

Fluorescence imaging using ICG has been used clinically to visualize the lymphatic drainage, liver cancer and bile duct anatomy in real time during surgery, and is beginning to be applied to laparoscopic surgery. In order to further enhance the sensitivity and specificity of intraoperative fluorescence imaging, we need to improve the imaging systems used for visualizing the fluorescence of ICG and also develop novel fluorescent agents that would enable cancer-specific identification of other hepatobiliary and pancreatic malignancies besides hepatocellular carcinoma.

Acknowledgements

This work was supported by grants from the Takeda Science Foundation, the Kanae Foundation for the Promotion of Medical Science, and the Ministry of Education, Culture, Sports, Science and Technology of Japan (No. 23689060).

References

1 Landsman ML, Kwant G, Mook GA, et al: Light-absorbing properties, stability, and spectral stabilization of indocyanine green. J Appl Physiol 1976;40:575–583.
2 Guyer DR, Puliafito CA, Monés JM, et al: Digital indocyanine-green angiography in chorioretinal disorders. Ophthalmology 1992;99:287–291.
3 Ogata F, Azuma R, Kikuchi M, et al: Novel lymphography using indocyanine green dye for near-infrared fluorescence labeling. Ann Plast Surg 2007;58:652–655.
4 Kitai T, Inomoto T, Miwa M, et al: Fluorescence navigation with indocyanine green for detecting sentinel lymph nodes in breast cancer. Breast Cancer 2005;12:211–215.
5 Kusano M, Tajima Y, Yamazaki K, et al: Sentinel node mapping guided by indocyanine green fluorescence imaging: a new method for sentinel node navigation surgery in gastrointestinal cancer. Dig Surg 2008;25:103–108.
6 Rubens FD, Ruel M, Fremes SE: A new and simplified method for coronary and graft imaging during CABG. Heart Surg Forum 2002;5:141–144.
7 Raabe A, Nakaji P, Beck J, et al: Prospective evaluation of surgical microscope-integrated intraoperative near-infrared indocyanine green videoangiography during aneurysm surgery. J Neurosurg 2005;103:982–989.
8 Kubota K, Kita J, Shimoda M, et al: Intraoperative assessment of reconstructed vessels in living-donor liver transplantation, using a novel fluorescence imaging technique. J Hepatobiliary Pancreat Surg 2006;13:100–104.
9 Mitsuhashi N, Kimura F, Shimizu H, et al: Usefulness of intraoperative fluorescence imaging to evaluate local anatomy in hepatobiliary surgery. J Hepatobiliary Pancreat Surg 2008;15:508–514.
10 Ishizawa T, Tamura S, Masuda K, et al: Intraoperative fluorescent cholangiography using indocyanine green: a biliary road map for safe surgery. J Am Coll Surg 2008;208:e1–e4.
11 Ishizawa T, Fukushima N, Shibahara J, et al: Real-time identification of liver cancers by using indocyanine green fluorescent imaging. Cancer 2009;115:2491–2504.
12 Gotoh K, Yamada T, Ishikawa O, et al: A novel image-guided surgery of hepatocellular carcinoma by indocyanine green fluorescence imaging navigation. J Surg Oncol 2009;100:75–79.
13 Yokoyama N, Otani T, Hashidate H, et al: Real-time detection of hepatic micrometastases from pancreatic cancer by intraoperative fluorescence imaging: preliminary results of a prospective study. Cancer 2012;118:2813–2819.
14 Ishizawa T, Bandai Y, Kokudo N: Fluorescent cholangiography using indocyanine green for laparoscopic cholecystectomy: an initial experience. Arch Surg 2009;144:381–382.

15 Ishizawa T, Bandai Y, Ijichi M, et al: Fluorescent cholangiography illuminating the biliary tree during laparoscopic cholecystectomy. Br J Surg 2010;97:1369–1377.
16 Ishizawa T, Kaneko J, Inoue Y, et al: Application of fluorescent cholangiography to single-incision laparoscopic cholecystectomy. Surg Endosc 2011;25:2631–2636.
17 Sherwinter DA: Identification of anomolous biliary anatomy using near-infrared cholangiography. J Gastrointest Surg 2012;16:1814–1815.
18 Giulianotti PC, Calatayud D, Milone L, et al: Fluorescence guidance for identification of the cystic duct-common bile duct junction: first experience in robotic surgery. Surg Endosc 2012;26:S353.
19 Buchs NN, Pugin F, Volonte F, et al: Intra-operative fluorescent cholangiography using indocyanine green for robotic single site cholecystectomy. Surg Endosc 2012;26:S443.
20 Ferraina P, Dip F, Lisandro A, et al: Safe cholecistectomy. Fluorescent cholangiography. Surg Endosc 2012;26:S443.
21 Goetz M, Deris I, Vieth M, et al: Near-infrared confocal imaging during mini-laparoscopy: a novel rigid endomicroscope with increased imaging plane depth. J Hepatol 2010;53:84–90.
22 Charlesworth P, Truscott TG: The use of 5-aminolevulinic acid (ALA) in photodynamic therapy (PDT). J Photochem Photobiol B 1993;18:99–100.
23 Hinnen P, de Rooij FW, van Velthuysen ML, et al: Biochemical basis of 5-aminolaevulinic acid-induced protoporphyrin IX accumulation: a study in patients with (pre)malignant lesions of the oesophagus. Br J Cancer 1998;78:679–682.
24 Stummer W, Stocker S, Wagner S, et al: Intraoperative detection of malignant gliomas by 5-aminolevulinic acid-induced porphyrin fluorescence. Neurosurgery 1998;42:518–525.
25 Kriegmair M, Stepp H, Steinbach P, et al: Fluorescence cystoscopy following intravesical instillation of 5-aminolevulinic acid: a new procedure with high sensitivity for detection of hardly visible urothelial neoplasias. Urol Int 1995;55:190–196.
26 Kishi K, Fujiwara Y, Yano M, et al: Staging laparoscopy using ALA-mediated photodynamic diagnosis improves the detection of peritoneal metastases in advanced gastric cancer. J Surg Oncol 2012;106:294–298.
27 Murayama Y, Harada Y, Imaizumi K, et al: Precise detection of lymph node metastases in mouse rectal cancer by using 5-aminolevulinic acid. Int J Cancer 2009;125:2256–2263.
28 Egger NG, Motamedi M, Pow-Sang M, et al: Accumulation of porphyrins in plasma and tissues of dogs after delta-aminolevulinic acid administration: implications for photodynamic therapy. Pharmacology 1996;52:362–370.
29 Figueiredo JL, Siegel C, Nahrendorf M, et al: Intraoperative near-infrared fluorescent cholangiography (NIRFC) in mouse models of bile duct injury. World J Surg 2010;34:336–343.
30 Ashitate Y, Stockdale A, Choi HS, et al: Real-time simultaneous near-infrared fluorescence imaging of bile duct and arterial anatomy. J Surg Res 2012;176:7–13.
31 Ogawa M, Kosaka N, Choyke PL, et al: In vivo molecular imaging of cancer with a quenching near-infrared fluorescent probe using conjugates of monoclonal antibodies and indocyanine green. Cancer Res 2009;69:1268–1272.
32 Metildi CA, Kaushal S, Lee C, et al: An LED light source and novel fluorophore combinations improve fluorescence laparoscopic detection of metastatic pancreatic cancer in orthotopic mouse models. J Am Coll Surg 2012;214:997–1007.
33 Urano Y, Sakabe M, Kosaka N, et al: Rapid cancer detection by topically spraying a γ-glutamyltranspeptidase-activated fluorescent probe. Sci Transl Med 2011;3:110–119.
34 Pompella A, De Tata V, Paolicchi A, et al: Expression of gamma-glutamyltransferase in cancer cells and its significance in drug resistance. Biochem Pharmacol 2006;71:231–238.
35 Aoki T, Yasuda, Shimizu Y, et al: Image-guided liver mapping using fluorescence navigation system with indocyanine green for anatomical hepatic resection. World J Surg 2008;32:1763–1767.
36 Uchiyama K, Ueno M, Ozawa S, et al: Combined intraoperative use of contrast-enhanced ultrasonography imaging using a sonazoid and fluorescence navigation system with indocyanine green during anatomical hepatectomy. Langenbecks Arch Surg 2011;396:1101–1107.
37 Kasuya K, Sugimoto K, Kyo B, et al: Ultrasonography-guided hepatic tumor resection using a real-time virtual sonography with indocyanine green navigation (with videos). J Hepatobiliary Pancreat Sci 2011;18:380–385.
38 Ishizawa T, Zuker NB, Kokudo N, Gayet B: Positive and negative staining of hepatic segments by use of fluorescent imaging techniques during laparoscopic hepatectomy. Arch Surg 2012;147:393–394.
39 Ishizawa T, Tamura S, Masuda K, et al: Intraoperative fluorescent cholangiography using indocyanine green: a biliary road map for safe recovery. J Am Coll Surg 2009;208:e1–e4.
40 Aoki T, Murakami M, Yasuda D, et al: Intraoperative fluorescent imaging using indocyanine green for liver mapping and cholangiography. J Hepatobiliary Pancreat Sci 2010;17:590–594.

41 Tagaya N, Shimodo M, Kato M, et al: Intraoperative exploration of biliary anatomy using fluorescence imaging of indocyanine green in experimental and clinical cholecystectomies. J Hepatobiliary Pancreat Sci 2010;17:595–600.
42 Sakaguchi T, Suzuki A, Unno N, et al: Bile leak test by indocyanine green fluorescence images after hepatectomy. Am J Surg 2010;200:e19–e23.
43 Mizuno S, Isaji S: Indocyanine green (ICG) fluorescence imaging-guided cholangiography for donor hepatectomy in living donor liver transplantation. Am J Transplant 2010;10:2725–2726.
44 Hutteman M, van der Vorst JR, Mieog JS, et al: Near-infrared fluorescence imaging in patients undergoing pancreaticoduodenectomy. Eur Surg Res 2011; 47:90–97.
45 Kaibori M, Ishizaki M, Matsui K, Kwon AH: Intraoperative indocyanine green fluorescent imaging for prevention of bile leakage after hepatic resection. Surgery 2011;150:91–98.
46 Kawaguchi Y, Ishizawa T, Masuda K, et al: Hepatobiliary surgery guided by a novel fluorescent imaging technique for visualizing hepatic arteries, bile ducts, and liver cancers on color images. J Am Coll Surg 2011;212:e33–e39.
47 Ishizawa T, Bandai Y, Harada N, et al: Indocyanine green-fluorescent imaging of hepatocellular carcinoma during laparoscopic hepatectomy: an initial experience. Asian J Endosc Surg 2010;3:42–45.
48 Ishizuka M, Nagata H, Takagi K, et al: Fluorescence imaging visualizes three sets of regional lymph nodes in patients with lower rectal cancer. Hepatogastroenterology 2012;59:1381–1384.
49 Satou S, Ishizawa T, Masuda K, et al: Indocyanine green fluorescent imaging for detecting extrahepatic metastasis of hepatocellular carcinoma. J Gastroenterol 2012, E-pub ahead of print.
50 Morita Y, Sakaguchi T, Unno N, et al: Detection of hepatocellular carcinomas with near-infrared fluorescence imaging using indocyanine green: its usefulness and limitation. Int J Clin Oncol 2011, E-pub ahead of print.
51 Kai K, Satoh S, Watanabe T, Endo Y: Evaluation of cholecystic venous flow using indocyanine green fluorescence angiography. J Hepatobiliary Pancreat Sci 2010;17:147–151.
52 Harada N, Ishizawa T, Muraoka A, et al: Fluorescence navigation hepatectomy by visualization of localized cholestasis from bile duct tumor infiltration. J Am Coll Surg 2010;210:e2–e6.
53 Hirono S, Tani M, Kawai M, et al: Identification of the lymphatic drainage pathways from the pancreatic head guided by indocyanine green fluorescence imaging during pancreaticoduodenectomy. Dig Surg 2012;29:132–139.
54 Kaneko J, Ishizawa T, Masuda K, et al: Indocyanine green reinjection technique for use in fluorescent angiography concomitant with cholangiography during laparoscopic cholecystectomy. Endosc Percutan Tech 2012;22:341–344.
55 Kawaguchi Y, Ishizawa T, Miyata Y, et al: Portal uptake function in veno-occlusive regions evaluated by real-time fluorescent imaging using indocyanine green. J Hepatol 2013;58:247–253.

Norihiro Kokudo, MD, PhD
Hepato-Biliary-Pancreatic Surgery Division, Department of Surgery
Graduate School of Medicine, The University of Tokyo
7-3-1 Hongo, Bunkyo-ku, Tokyo 113-8655 (Japan)
E-Mail KOKUDO-2SU@h.u-tokyo.ac.jp

Kokudo N, Ishizawa T (eds): Fluorescent Imaging: Treatment of Hepatobiliary and Pancreatic Diseases.
Front Gastrointest Res. Basel, Karger, 2013, vol 31, pp 10–17 (DOI: 10.1159/000348601)

Identification of Hepatocellular Carcinoma

Takeaki Ishizawa · Norihiro Kokudo

Hepato-Biliary-Pancreatic Surgery Division, Department of Surgery, Graduate School of Medicine,
The University of Tokyo, Tokyo, Japan

Abstract

Fluorescence imaging using indocyanine green (ICG) enables highly sensitive identification of hepatocellular carcinoma (HCC) by allowing visualization of impaired biliary excretion of ICG in differentiated HCC tissues and/or in noncancerous liver parenchyma around the tumor. In this technique, ICG is administered intravenously at the dose of 0.5 mg/kg for routine liver function testing within 2 weeks prior to surgery. Intraoperatively, liver cancer can be easily identified by fluorescence imaging of the liver surface prior to resection and on the resected specimen. Intraoperative ICG fluorescence imaging is useful for detecting superficially located small HCCs and confirming that these lesions have been removed with sufficient surgical margins. The present technique also enables identification of new lesions of HCC that have not been diagnosed preoperatively; however, additional resection should be considered only after re-evaluation by visual inspection and palpation or intraoperative ultrasonography because the positive predictive values of such newly detected lesions are 50% or lower, especially when the ICG is administered on the day before the surgery in patients with liver cirrhosis.

In 2007, we developed a fluorescence imaging technique for intraoperative cholangiography using intrabiliary injection of indocyanine green (ICG) [1]. While developing this technique, we noticed that cancerous tissues on the liver surface emitted their own fluorescence even before the intraoperative administration of ICG for cholangiography. Actually, in all the patients at our department, ICG is administered intravenously before surgery in order to measure the ICG retention rate at 15 min as a routine liver function test. Thus, it was assumed that the intraoperative visualization of liver cancer by ICG fluorescence imaging was caused by accumulation of the ICG injected intravenously prior to the surgery in cancerous tissues and/or surrounding noncancerous liver tissues at the time of surgery. Then, a prospective clinical study was initiated to evaluate the efficacy of fluorescence imaging utilizing preoperatively injected ICG to detect liver cancer during surgery [2]. Here, we focus on the mechanistic background and clinical applications of intraoperative ICG fluorescence imaging of hepatocellular carcinoma (HCC). Other chapters in this volume detail the use of the ICG fluorescence imaging technique for the identification of metastatic liver cancer during surgery.

Principle of Indocyanine Green Fluorescence Imaging of Hepatocellular Cancer

Fluorescence imaging of liver cancer using preoperative intravenous administration of ICG is based on the fact that ICG is exclusively excreted into the bile and emits fluorescence that peaks at about 840 nm when protein-bound ICG is exposed to an excitation light in the range of 750–810 nm [3]. Because visualization at this wavelength is scarcely affected due to absorption by hemoglobin or water, biological structures that contain ICG can be visualized through tissue thicknesses of 5–10 mm with the use of an appropriate filter and a camera that is sensitive in the infrared region. On the other hand, a certain pathological type of HCC, termed 'green hepatoma', is known to retain the ability to produce bile. Furthermore, previous studies of delayed magnetic resonance imaging obtained 10–24 h after the administration of a contrast material excreted via bile suggested the presence of impaired bile excretion in HCC tissues as well as in noncancerous liver parenchyma surrounding the tumor, resulting in hyperenhancement of well-differentiated HCCs and rim enhancement of metastatic liver cancer [4–7]. Based on the above findings, we developed an intraoperative ICG fluorescence imaging technique aimed at visualizing liver cancer on the liver surface during surgery or on resected specimens based on the impaired biliary excretion in HCC tissues and in the noncancerous liver parenchyma around the tumor [2].

In our previous series consisting of 37 patients with HCC and 12 patients with colorectal liver metastasis, fluorescence imaging following preoperative intravenous administration of ICG at the dose of 0.5 mg/kg identified all of the microscopically confirmed HCCs (n = 63) and colorectal liver metastases (n = 28) on the cut surfaces of the resected specimens. The fluorescence patterns of these tumors were classifiable into the total fluorescence type (all of the cancer tissues showed uniform fluorescence), partial fluorescence type (a part of the cancer tissues showed fluorescence) and rim fluorescence type (the cancer tissues were negative for fluorescence, but the surrounding liver parenchyma showed fluorescence; fig. 1) [2, 8]. The fluorescence patterns were closely associated with the characteristics of the liver cancers: the total fluorescence-type tumors included all of the well-differentiated HCCs, while the rim fluorescence-type tumors consisted of only poorly differentiated HCCs and colorectal liver metastases. Furthermore, fluorescence microscopy confirmed the presence of fluorescence in the cytoplasm and pseudoglands of the HCC cells and in the noncancerous liver parenchyma surrounding the poorly differentiated HCCs and metastases (fig. 2).

These results are consistent with the previously proposed mechanism of ICG accumulation in cancerous tissues and/or noncancerous liver parenchyma around the tumor. Such pharmacokinetics of ICG in the liver involving HCC may be proven by

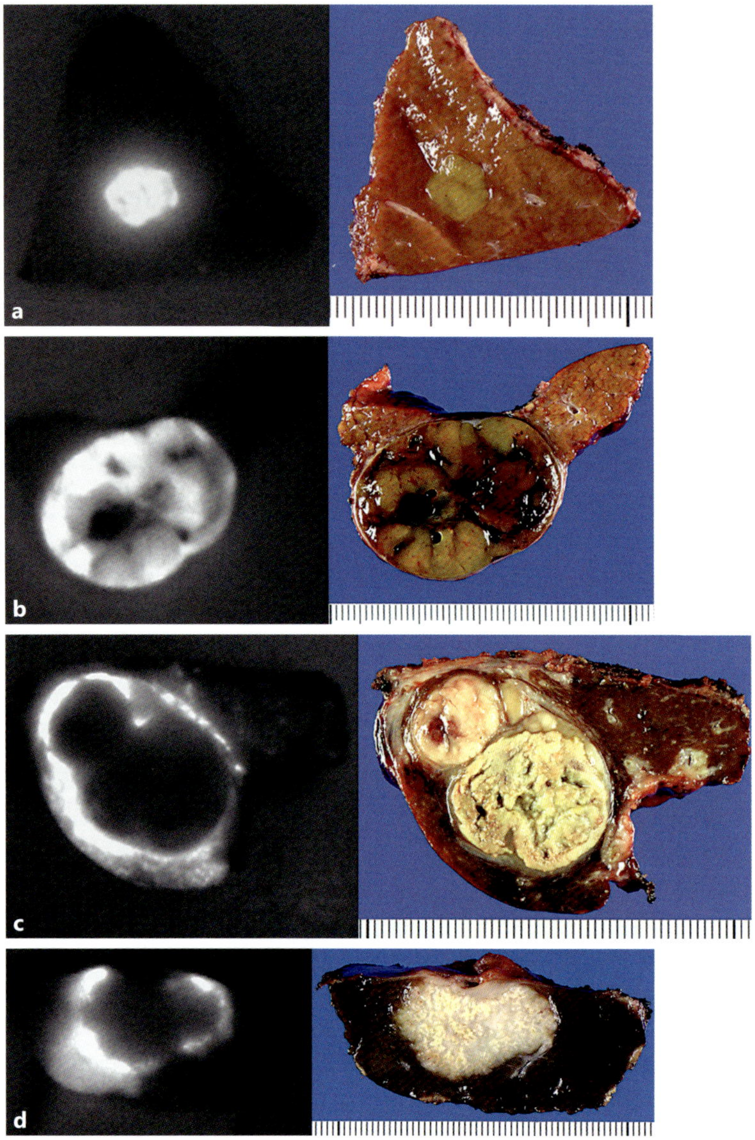

Fig. 1. Fluorescence patterns of liver cancers on cut surfaces of the liver (left) and their gross appearances (right) [8]. **a** Total fluorescence type (well-differentiated HCC, 7 mm in diameter). **b** Partial fluorescence type (moderately differentiated HCC, 35 mm in diameter). **c** Rim fluorescence type (poorly differentiated HCC, 30 mm in diameter). **d** Rim fluorescence type (metastasis of colorectal cancer, 25 mm in diameter).

gene expression analysis and immunohistochemical staining, as used in the previous study conducted to reveal the background of magnetic resonance imaging of HCC with gadolinium ethoxybenzyl diethylenetriamine pentaacetic acid [9]. Our preliminary results suggested that the expression levels of portal uptake transporters of ICG (organic anion-transporting polypeptides and Na^+/taurocholate cotransporting poly-

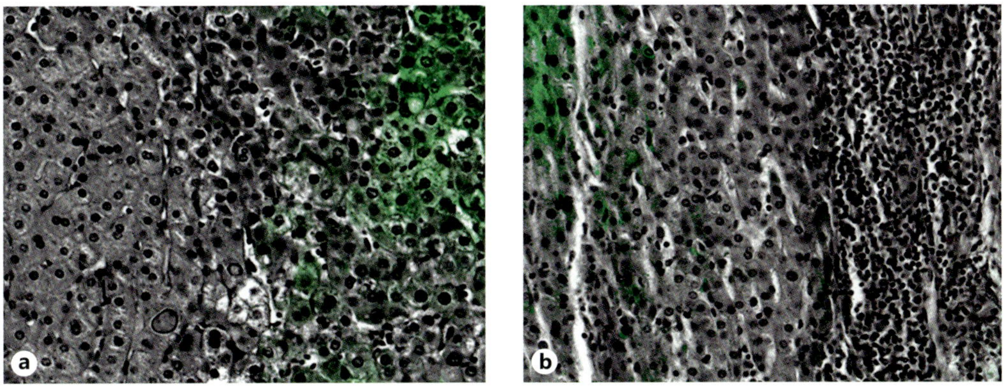

Fig. 2. Fluorescence microscopy. Fluorescence microscopy reveals that fluorescence of ICG (indicated in green) exists in cancerous tissues of well-differentiated HCC (**a**) and in noncancerous liver parenchyma around the tumor in poorly differentiated HCC (**b**).

peptide [10]) are well-preserved in HCCs showing fluorescence of ICG in the cancerous tissues as compared with the impaired gene expression levels in the cancerous tissues of rim fluorescence-type HCCs (unpubl. data).

Actually, the fluorescence imaging technique using ICG to identify liver cancer was included in a patent obtained by a group at the University of Rochester (WO 2008/043101 A2). Although there have been no detailed articles concerning liver cancer imaging, except for a recent article on ICG fluorescence imaging of renal cancer [11], their method is probably not based on the disordered biliary excretion of ICG, but on the difference in hemodynamics between cancerous tissues and noncancerous liver parenchyma that may occur in the earlier phase after intravenous administration of ICG.

Advantages and Limitations of the Use of Indocyanine Green

The major advantage of ICG fluorescence imaging is its sensitivity and feasibility: once the ICG retention test has been performed within 2 weeks prior to the surgery, surgeons can obtain fluorescence images of the liver cancer with a commercially available small imaging system at any time during the surgical procedures in order to detect cancerous tissues on the liver surface before resection or on the resected liver specimens. Although the ICG retention rate at 15 min has not been widely used as a preoperative liver function test in Western countries, this test is practically the only way to estimate the acceptable limit of liver volume to be removed in each patient [12]. Especially in liver resection for patients with background liver disease, it is strongly recommended that the ICG retention rate at 15 min be evaluated not only for intraoperative ICG fluorescence imaging of liver cancer, but also to ensure the safety of liver resection [13].

In contrast, it should be noted that when 0.5 mg/kg of ICG is administered intravenously for a liver function test on the day before surgery, washout from the noncancerous liver parenchyma is inadequate and there may be many false-positive nodules; the poorer the liver function, the more marked this tendency [2]. Further studies are needed to determine the optimal interval between ICG injection and surgery on the basis of the patient's liver function. Moreover, this technique does not use a cancer-specific antigen-antibody reaction. Instead, it just allows visualization of the impaired bile excretion in HCC tissues and/or noncancerous liver tissues around the tumor. Thus, benign lesions, such as regenerating nodules, bile duct proliferation and expanding liver cysts, may also exhibit fluorescence if there is delayed bile excretion. In fact, in previous reports, 40–50% of the lesions newly identified by fluorescence imaging during surgery were pathologically proven to be noncancerous lesions [2, 14, 15]. Even when new lesions are detected by ICG fluorescence imaging during surgery, additional resection should be considered only after the lesions have also been confirmed to be cancerous by inspection and palpation, and/or by an intraoperative ultrasonography.

Clinical Application of Indocyanine Green Fluorescence Imaging

Considering the advantages and limitations of ICG fluorescence imaging for liver cancer, its major expected roles in liver resection for HCC are to identify: (1) peripherally located, but invisible HCC diagnosed preoperatively, (2) new lesions to be considered for additional resection, (3) HCC tissues left on the raw surface of the liver after resection, and (4) small HCCs on the resected specimens.

In liver resection for HCC, especially during repeated resection for recurrence, surgeons sometimes encounter difficulty in detecting superficially located small tumors that need to be removed. This is because HCC tissues are often not hard enough to palpate and intraoperative ultrasonography has limitations in visualizing small lesions located just beneath the liver surface. In such instances, ICG fluorescence imaging is useful for visualizing the lesions to be resected (fig. 3a). During liver resection for advanced HCC with infiltration of the portal pedicle, fluorescence imaging delineates cholestatic regions on the liver surface, which can be used as a guide for determination of the hepatic transection line (fig. 3b) [16].

In previous series, approximately 10% of all pathologically diagnosed HCCs were grossly unidentifiable and detected by using intraoperative ICG fluorescence imaging on the resected specimens [2, 14, 15]. This technique not only increases the accuracy of pathological diagnosis, especially in the case of small HCCs with an indistinct margin (early HCC), but also enhances the resectability of HCC. For example, ICG fluorescence imaging can be used to confirm surgical margins during surgery when the tumor boundary is unclear by gross examination of the cut surfaces of resected specimens (fig. 3c). If the surgical margins are insufficient on fluorescence images on the

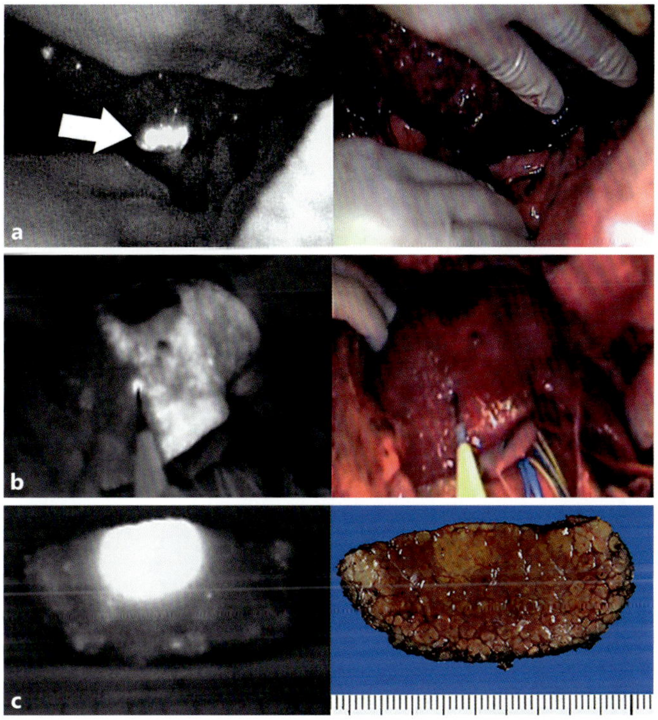

Fig. 3. Applications of ICG fluorescence imaging during liver resection for HCC. **a** Fluorescence imaging identifies HCC (arrow) on the irregular liver surface with cirrhosis. **b** Fluorescence imaging clearly delineates the cholestatic hepatic regions caused by bile duct invasion of HCC located in the right paramedian sector. The demarcation is marked by electrocautery as the potential hepatic transection line. **c** Fluorescence imaging on the resected specimen is used in the operation room to confirm the surgical margin after resection of HCC with an indistinct margin on gross examination.

resected specimen, fluorescence images of the raw surfaces of the remnant liver should be obtained to confirm the presence or absence of the remaining cancerous tissues. ICG fluorescence imaging can also be applied to identification of extrahepatic metastasis of HCCs utilizing bile production by metastatic lesions [17].

Future Perspectives

With the advent of surgical techniques and instruments, laparoscopic liver resection has recently been able to offer the possibility of anatomic segmentectomy [18, 19], which can provide oncological benefit for patients with HCC [20]. In order to enhance the safety and accuracy of minimally invasive surgical treatment for HCC, it is essential to improve the quality of laparoscopic and robotic fluorescence imaging systems [21, 22] to overcome the limitations of laparoscopic surgery in intraoperative diagnosis resulting from lack of palpation. Simultaneous visualization of ICG-specific fluorescent signals on color images may further enhance the feasibility of fluorescence imaging during liver resection [23]. Although fluorescence imaging is limited concerning its ability to allow visualization of deeply located liver cancers, photoacoustic imaging techniques [24] using ICG may have the potential to overcome this problem.

One of the outstanding characteristics of ICG fluorescence imaging of HCC is that it allows high lesion-to-background contrast for well- or moderately differentiated HCC (median: 2.6-fold, range: 0.6–16.6; unpubl. data) as compared to fluorescence imaging using ICG for other kinds of cancer tissues (up to twofold) [25, 26]. This suggests that a novel photodynamic therapy for HCC may be realized by utilizing the ICG accumulated in HCC tissues for prolonged periods of time following intravenous administration as a photosensitive substance.

Conclusion

Intraoperative ICG fluorescence imaging is quite simple and enables highly sensitive identification of HCC by allowing visualization of the impaired biliary excretion of ICG in HCC tissues and/or in noncancerous liver parenchyma. In order to fully utilize ICG fluorescence imaging in liver resection, it is important to understand the simple mechanistic background of this technique – *there is fluorescence where there is bile.*

Acknowledgements

This work was supported by grants from the Takeda Science Foundation, the Kanae Foundation for the Promotion of Medical Science, and the Ministry of Education, Culture, Sports, Science and Technology of Japan (No. 23689060).

References

1 Ishizawa T, Tamura S, Masuda K, et al: Intraoperative fluorescent cholangiography using indocyanine green: a biliary road map for safe surgery. J Am Coll Surg 2008;208:e1–e4.
2 Ishizawa T, Fukushima N, Shibahara J, et al: Real-time identification of liver cancers by using indocyanine green fluorescent imaging. Cancer 2009;115: 2491–2504.
3 Landsman ML, Kwant G, Mook GA, et al: Light-absorbing properties, stability, and spectral stabilization of indocyanine green. J Appl Physiol 1976;40: 575–583.
4 Ni Y, Marchal G, Yu J, et al: Experimental liver cancers: Mn-DPDP-enhanced rims in MR-microangiographic-histologic correlation study. Radiology 1993;188:45–51.
5 Coffin CM, Diche T, Mahfouz A, et al: Benign and malignant hepatocellular tumors: evaluation of tumoral enhancement after mangafodipir trisodium injection on MR imaging. Eur Radiol1999;9:444–449.
6 Wang DB, Zhou KR, Zeng MS, et al: Mn-DPDP-enhanced 24-h delayed-scan MRI of hepatocellular carcinoma is correlated with histology. Eur Radiol 2004;14:743–745.
7 Chung JJ, Kim MJ, Kim KW: Mangafodipir trisodiumenhanced MRI for the detection and characterization of focal hepatic lesions: is delayed imaging useful? J Magn Reson Imaging 2006;23:706–711.
8 Ishizawa T, Harada N, Muraoka A, et al: Scientific basis and clinical application of ICG fluorescence imaging: hepatobiliary cancer. Open Surg Oncol J 2010;2:31–36.
9 Kitao A, Zen Y, Matsui O, et al: Hepatocellular carcinoma: signal intensity at gadoxetic acid-enhanced MR Imaging – correlation with molecular transporters and histopathologic features. Radiology 2010; 256:817–826.
10 de Graaf W, Häusler S, Heger M, et al: Transporters involved in the hepatic uptake of (99m)Tc-mebrofenin and indocyanine green. J Hepatol 2011;54: 738–745.

11 Tobis S, Knopf J, Silvers C, et al: Near infrared fluorescence imaging with robotic assisted laparoscopic partial nephrectomy: initial clinical experience for renal cortical tumors. J Urol 2011;186:47–52.
12 Makuuchi M, Kosuge T, Takayama T, et al: Surgery for small liver cancers. Semin Surg Oncol 1993;9: 298–304.
13 Ishizawa T, Hasegawa K, Aoki T, et al: Neither multiple tumors nor portal hypertension are surgical contraindications for hepatocellular carcinoma. Gastroenterology 2008;134:1908–1916.
14 Gotoh K, Yamada T, Ishikawa O, et al: A novel image-guided surgery of hepatocellular carcinoma by indocyanine green fluorescence imaging navigation. J Surg Oncol 2009;100:75–79.
15 Ishizuka M, Kubota K, Kita J, et al: Intraoperative observation using a fluorescence imaging instrument during hepatic resection for liver metastasis from colorectal cancer. Hepatogastroenterology 2012;59:90–92.
16 Harada N, Ishizawa T, Muraoka A, et al: Fluorescence navigation hepatectomy by visualization of localized cholestasis from bile duct tumor infiltration. J Am Coll Surg 2010;210:e2–e6.
17 Satou S, Ishizawa T, Kokudo N, et al: Indocyanine green fluorescent imaging for detecting extrahepatic metastasis of hepatocellular carcinoma. J Gastroenterol 2012, E-pub ahead of print.
18 Ishizawa T, Gumbs AA, Kokudo N, Gayet B: Laparoscopic segmentectomy of the liver: from segment I to VIII. Ann Surg 2012;256:959–964.
19 Ishizawa T, Zuker NB, Kokudo N, Gayet B: Positive and negative staining of hepatic segments by use of fluorescent imaging techniques during laparoscopic hepatectomy. Arch Surg 2012;147:393–394.
20 Hasegawa K, Kokudo N, Imamura H, et al: Prognostic impact of anatomic resection for hepatocellular carcinoma. Ann Surg 2005;242:252–259.
21 Ishizawa T, Bandai Y, Ijichi M, et al: Fluorescent cholangiography illuminating the biliary tree during laparoscopic cholecystectomy. Br J Surg 2010;97: 1369–1377.
22 Ishizawa T, Bandai Y, Harada N, et al: Indocyanine green-fluorescent imaging of hepatocellular carcinoma during laparoscopic hepatectomy: an initial experience. Asian J Endosc Surg 2010;3:42–45.
23 Kawaguchi Y, Ishizawa T, Masuda K, et al: Hepatobiliary surgery guided by a novel fluorescent imaging technique for visualizing hepatic arteries, bile ducts, and liver cancers on color images. J Am Coll Surg 2011;212:e33–e39.
24 Wang LV: Multiscale photoacoustic microscopy and computed tomography. Nat Photonics 2009;3:503–509.
25 Thayer D, Unlu MB, Lin Y, et al: Dual-contrast dynamic MRI-DOT for small animal imaging. Technol Cancer Res Treat 2010;9:61–70.
26 Kim TH, Mount CW, Dulken BW, et al: Filamentous, mixed micelles of triblock copolymers enhance tumor localization of indocyanine green in a murine xenograft model. Mol Pharm 2012;9:135–143.

Norihiro Kokudo, MD, PhD
Hepato-Biliary-Pancreatic Surgery Division, Department of Surgery
Graduate School of Medicine, The University of Tokyo
7-3-1 Hongo, Bunkyo-ku, Tokyo 113-8655 (Japan)
E-Mail KOKUDO-2SU@h.u-tokyo.ac.jp

Kokudo N, Ishizawa T (eds): Fluorescent Imaging: Treatment of Hepatobiliary and Pancreatic Diseases.
Front Gastrointest Res. Basel, Karger, 2013, vol 31, pp 18–24 (DOI: 10.1159/000350038)

Identification of Metastatic Liver Cancer

Chetana Lim[a] · Eric Vibert[b]

[a] AP-HP, Hôpital Henri Mondor, Créteil, and [b] AP-HP, Hôpital Paul Brousse, Villejuif, France

Abstract

Indocyanine green (ICG) is a vital dye excreted in bile duct that can be trapped around or into liver tumor. The presence of the dye at the surface of the liver can be detected using an infrared ICG camera. It is now possible to identify in real time liver tumors during hepatectomy using this novel fluorescence imaging technique. Intraoperative ICG fluorescence imaging usually identifies colorectal liver metastases as rim-fluorescing lesions with a low lesion-to-liver contrast. However, one of the main limitations of this technique may be its limited ability to detect deep lesions. In this chapter, we report our single-center experience with preliminary results following intraoperative detection of subcapsular tumors in 32 patients with colorectal liver metastases and perform a systematic review of published studies.

Liver resection offers a chance of a cure in selected patients with colorectal liver metastases. However, surgery is possible only if all metastatic lesions can be completely resected (R0 resection) and if the quality and volume of the remnant liver parenchyma are acceptable [1]. Several independent predictors of survival are well known such as the number of lesions, lymph node-positive primary tumors, poorly differentiated primary tumors, extrahepatic disease, tumor size, carcinoembryonic antigen levels and positive resection margins; however, none of these represents an absolute contraindication [2, 3]. In particular, a large number of liver metastases should not be considered as a contraindication to curative resection [4].

Therefore, to achieve curative surgery, precise staging of the extent of the disease and intraoperative identification of all lesions are required. For evaluation of the extent of the liver disease, contrast-enhanced computed tomography (CT) and/or magnetic resonance imaging (MRI) are recommended [5]. Intraoperative ultrasonography (IOUS) and (recently) contrast-enhanced IOUS (CE-IOUS) are used for intraoperative identification of liver tumors. Several studies have shown that CE-IOUS can find more lesions than conventional IOUS [6] and was more sensitive than a CT scan and/or MRI in detecting liver metastases [7]. However, the intraoperative identification of small tumors remains a major concern as 3–17% of hepatocellular carcinoma

Table 1. Fluorescence pattern of liver metastases

Authors/ country/ref.	Typical features of fluorescence pattern of liver metastases		Timing of ICG injection	Limitations
	before resection	resected specimen		
Uchiyama et al. Japan [12]	rim fluorescence	rim fluorescence	2 weeks before surgery	additional features of fluorescence pattern for liver metastases (uniform or partial fluorescent signals)
Ishizawa et al. Japan [8]	rim fluorescence	rim fluorescence	1–14 days before surgery	cirrhosis (increased ICG retention rate) patients who had received the ICG injection within 24 h
Vibert et al. France (unpubl. data)	rim fluorescence	rim fluorescence	14 h before surgery	area of liver with portal vein embolization

and liver metastases can be detected only by microscopic examination [8]. Also, chemotherapy can result in images showing complete disappearance of preoperatively detected liver metastases [9].

Recently it has been shown that indocyanine green (ICG) fluorescence imaging has great potential to improve the accuracy of intraoperative identification of liver cancers during hepatectomy. Liver tumors can be visualized using an infrared camera system, due to the accumulation of preoperatively injected ICG inside or around the tumor cells.

The aim of this chapter is to describe the clinical role of ICG fluorescence imaging in intraoperative diagnosis of colorectal liver metastases and to report our single-center results.

Features of Liver Metastases on Indocyanine Green Fluorescence Imaging

Intraoperative ICG fluorescence imaging usually identifies colorectal liver metastases as rim-fluorescing lesions with a low lesion-to-liver contrast (table 1). The fluorescent peripheral rim corresponds to the nontumorous liver parenchyma surrounding the tumor, and the nonfluorescent area in the center of the ring represents the tumor mass (fig. 1). Because of biliary excretion disorders (due to compression by the tumor), ICG injection is retained selectively by the hepatic cells surrounding the metastases and provides rim fluorescence. These features are the same as those displayed during MRI using liver-specific contrast medium such as Gd-EOB-DTPA [10, 11]. However, it is subject to variations as liver metastases may show variable fluorescent patterns such as uniform or partial fluorescing enhancement. It does not seem to be dependent on the tumor grade or the size of the lesions.

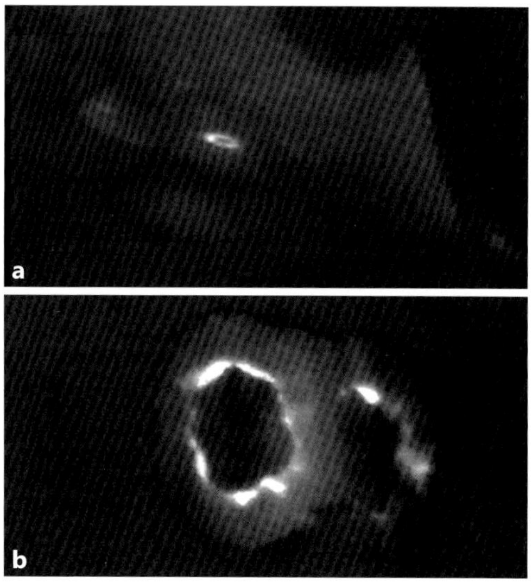

Fig. 1. Liver tumor in the left liver that was not palpable unless observed using the fluorescence imaging technique. **a** Intraoperative fluorescence imaging technique identified a bright rim fluorescent signal on the liver surface. **b** A metastatic lesion was confirmed by histological analysis.

The optimal time to scan for all liver metastases is 2–14 days after ICG injection. This is the time when the contrast between the fluorescent normal liver surrounding the tumor and the nonfluorescent metastases is most pronounced to obtain an optimal lesion-to-liver contrast. Indeed, the signal intensity of the nontumorous liver parenchyma, particularly in patients with an elevated ICG retention rate (with an underlying liver disease) and in those who had received the ICG injection within 24 h before surgery, could interfere with that of the metastases.

The Paul Brousse Experience

Between November 2010 and June 2012, 32 patients underwent open hepatectomy for colorectal liver metastases at the Centre Hepato-Biliaire (Villejuif, France). In our center, an ICG test is routinely used to assess liver function before liver resection and is intravenously injected the day before surgery at a dose of 0.5 mg/kg (around 14 h before surgery). All patients had an ICG retention rate at 15 min within the normal range.

During surgery, the liver was first mobilized and evaluated by bimanual palpation and IOUS to assess the number and location of metastases. Then, the liver surface was screened by the fluorescence imaging system (PDE; Hamamatsu Photonics, Hamamatsu, Japan) before resection. All newly detected lesions were assessed by manual palpation and then resected.

ICG fluorescence imaging detected more subcapsular liver metastases than manual palpation and IOUS (table 2). Additional liver metastases were found in 13% of cases (n = 4 patients), which resulted in the modification of the surgical plans in all cases (additional limited hepatectomies). Of these 4 patients, 3 had malignant lesions according

Table 2. Studies investigating the clinical significance of intraoperative ICG fluorescence imaging

Authors/ date/ref.	Country	patients, n	Reference standard used	Type of analysis	Sensitivity		Predictive positive value	
					conventional imaging	ICG of the liver surface before resection	conventional imaging	ICG of the liver surface before resection
Ishizawa et al. 2009 [8]	Japan	12[1]	histological examination of resected specimen	lesion-by-lesion	IOUS 100%	100%	–	100%
Uchiyama et al. 2010 [12]	Japan	32	histological examination of resected specimen	lesion-by-lesion	combined CT/MRI 88.5%	98.1%	combined CT/MRI 95.5%	96.3%
Vibert et al. (unpubl. data)	France	32	histological examination of resected specimen	patient-by-patient	IOUS missed metastatic lesions in 3 patients	found additional lesions in 4 patients (true positive in 3 cases and false positive in 1 case)	–	–

[1] 6 patients were assessed by ICG fluorescence imaging.

to the histopathological examination and 1 had a necrotic lesion. Additional liver metastases were all infracentimetric and were revealed as a small deposit surrounded by a fluorescent ring. The necrotic lesion was millimetric and was revealed as a little spot as seen in hepatocellular carcinoma (see Ishizawa and Kokudo [this vol., pp 1–9]). The latter lesion was intraoperatively considered as malignant because the manual palpation was positive as in the other 3 cases. Retrospectively, the question still remains whether that lesion was initially a tumor that showed a complete response after chemotherapy.

Literature Review

The effectiveness of intraoperative ICG fluorescence imaging in patients with colorectal liver metastases has been shown only by two published studies. Ishizawa et al. [8] was the first to show that ICG fluorescence imaging can be used to detect hepatocellular carcinoma and metastatic lesions based on their tumorous and nontumorous fluorescence, respectively. In this study, all microscopically confirmed liver metastases (n = 28 lesions) were previously identified by ICG fluorescence imaging of both liver surface and resected specimens. For hepatocellular carcinoma, particularly well- or moderately differentiated cancer tissues, tumors appear as uniformly and highly fluorescing lesions (fluorescence originated in the cytoplasm of hepatocellular carci-

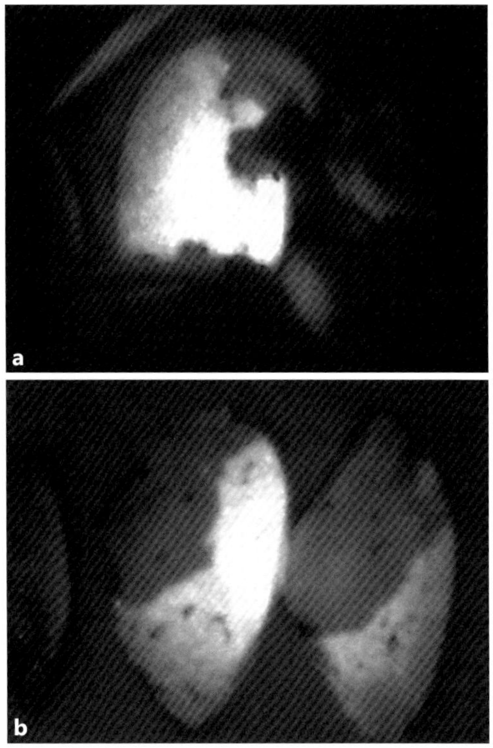

Fig. 2. Intraoperative ICG fluorescence image of the right liver after portal vein embolization. **a** Intraoperative findings revealed a high signal intensity located in the right embolized liver lobe. **b** On the resected specimen, fluorescence imaging detected the area corresponding to the area of liver with portal vein embolization.

noma cells), while poorly differentiated hepatocellular carcinoma and colorectal liver metastases display rim fluorescence (fluorescence originates from the surrounding nontumorous liver parenchyma which is compressed by the tumor).

Uchiyama et al. [12] reported that 4 additional lesions, in which 2 were metastatic lesions, were visualized using ICG fluorescence imaging. These lesions were not detected by CT scan, MRI or intraoperative CE-IOUS. All these lesions were located at the liver surface. However, they also reported that metastatic lesions might show a variable fluorescence pattern such as complete fluorescence (5/27 lesions), partial fluorescence (4/27 lesions) and ring fluorescence (18/27 lesions). Additionally, combined IOUS/ICG fluorescence imaging was compared with preoperative combined CT scan/MRI in this study [12], which showed a further value for ICG fluorescence imaging (table 2).

Limitations of Indocyanine Green Fluorescence Imaging of the Liver

ICG fluorescence imaging has limited ability to detect deep lesions. A tumor can only be visualized if it is located on the surface of the liver. Ishizawa et al. [8] described that a lesion located at a depth of more than 8 mm from the liver surface, irrespective of the size, was missed by this procedure. In our experience, it was not possible to assess the presence of suspected lesions in the embolized part of the liver after portal vein embolization (fig. 2). Moreover, it may be difficult to differentiate suspected lesions from the surrounding liver parenchyma when the signal intensity of the surrounding liver parenchyma is high. This has been the case in patients with an underlying liver disease (thus with an increased ICG retention rate) and in patients who had received the ICG injection within 8 h before surgery.

Current Situations and Perspectives

ICG fluorescence imaging techniques have been applied to hepatobiliary surgery in Japan for the last few years, but it is not commonly used in Western countries. These techniques enable real-time identification of new liver tumors. However, this imaging system might not replace all of the roles of the conventional IOUS and CE-IOUS because of the limited tissue penetration ability of ICG fluorescence up to 5 mm and various factors affecting fluorescence imaging [13].

One of the main advantages of this imaging system is that fluorescence imaging can be performed simply and quickly in a real-time setting. Once ICG is administered in the days prior to surgery, fluorescence images can be obtained by simply placing the camera imaging head on the liver surface. One major concern may be its safety. The ICG clearance test is widely used in many hepatobiliary centers in Asia to evaluate liver function before resection. The low risk after intravenous injection of adverse events has recently been clearly evaluated [14].

Besides its ability to detect small and unidentifiable liver metastases, this novel real-time imaging technique appears to be useful for detecting endobiliary metastases because, if present, anatomical resection rather than partial resection is required. From an oncological point of view, it may be promising in detecting microscopic residual cancerous tissues on the raw surface of the remnant liver after resection. Finally, this imaging technique may become an additional tool for identifying liver metastases during laparoscopic liver resection in which surgeons cannot palpate the liver surface.

Conclusion

For now, ICG fluorescence imaging should remain a complement to conventional imaging techniques, such as IOUS or CE-IOUS during open or laparoscopic liver resection. This imaging system has great potential for the detection of primary and metastatic liver malignancies, and thus improving intraoperative imaging assessment of the liver. Further clinical studies comparing preoperative CT scan/MRI versus ICG fluorescence imaging and CE-IOUS versus ICG fluorescence imaging, and long-term outcome studies for the assessment of liver metastases are needed to determine its true value in clinical practice

References

1 Clavien PA, Petrowsky H, DeOliveira ML, Graf R: Strategies for safer liver surgery and partial liver transplantation. N Engl J Med 2007;356:1545–1559.

2 Adam R, Da Gramont A, Figueras J, et al: The oncosurgery approach to managing liver metastases from colorectal cancer: a multidisciplinary international consensus. Oncologist 2012;17:1225–1239.

3 Rees M, Tekkis PP, Welsh FK, O'Rourke T, John TG: Evaluation of long-term survival after hepatic resection for metastatic colorectal cancer: a multifactorial model of 929 patients. Ann Surg 2008;247:125–135.

4 Bolton JS, Fuhrman GM: Survival after resection of multiple bilobar hepatic metastases from colorectal carcinoma. Ann Surg 2000;231:743–751.

5 Adams RB, Aloia TA, Loyer E, et al: Selection for hepatic resection of colorectal liver metastases: expert consensus statement. HPB (Oxford) 2012;15:91–103.

6 Chami L, Lassau N, Malka D, et al: Benefits of contrast-enhanced sonography for the detection of liver lesions: comparison with histologic findings. AJR Am J Roentgenol 2008;190:683–690.

7 Leen E, Cecotti P, Moug SJ, et al: Potential value of contrast-enhanced intraoperative ultrasonography during partial hepatectomy for metastases: an essential investigation before resection? Ann Surg 2006; 243:236–240.

8 Ishizawa T, Fukushima N, Shibahara J, et al: Realtime identification of liver cancers by using indocyanine green fluorescent imaging. Cancer 2009;115: 2491–2504.

9 Benoist S, Brouquet A, Penna C, et al: Complete response of colorectal liver metastases after chemotherapy: does it mean cure? J Clin Oncol 2006;24: 3939–3945.

10 Coffin CM, Diche T, Mahfouz A, et al: Benign and malignant hepatocellular tumors: evaluation of tumoral enhancement after mangafodipir trisodium injection on MR imaging. Eur Radiol 1999;9:444–449.

11 Chung JJ, Kim MJ, Kim KW: Mangafodipir trisodium-enhanced MRI for the detection and characterization of focal hepatic lesions: is delayed imaging useful? J Magn Reson Imaging 2006;23:706–711.

12 Uchiyama K, Ueno M, Ozawa S, et al: Combined use of contrast-enhanced intraoperative ultrasonography and a fluorescence navigation system for identifying hepatic metastases. World J Surg 2010;34: 2953–2959.

13 Morita Y, Sakaguchi T, Unno N, et al: Detection of hepatocellular carcinomas with near-infrared fluorescence imaging using indocyanine green: its usefulness and limitation. Int J Clin Oncol 2011, E-pub ahead of print.

14 Cherrick GR, Stein SW, Leevy CM, Davidson CS: Indocyanine green: observations on its physical properties, plasma decay, and hepatic extraction. J Clin Invest 1960;39:592–600.

Dr. Eric Vibert
Centre Hépato-Biliaire, Hôpital Paul Brousse-Assistance Publique-Hôpitaux de Paris
Faculté de Médecine, Université Paris Kremlin-Bicètre
12 Avenue Paul Vaillant Couturier, FR–94804 Villejuif (France)
E-Mail eric.vibert.pbr@gmail.com

Kokudo N, Ishizawa T (eds): Fluorescent Imaging: Treatment of Hepatobiliary and Pancreatic Diseases.
Front Gastrointest Res. Basel, Karger, 2013, vol 31, pp 25–32 (DOI: 10.1159/000348603)

Identification of Occult Liver Metastases

Naoyuki Yokoyama · Tetsuya Otani

Department of Digestive Surgery, Niigata City General Hospital, Niigata, Japan

Abstract

Background /Aim: Assessment of hepatic metastases is of major importance in the treatment of digestive tract cancers. Even with advanced clinical imaging modalities, extremely small hepatic micrometastases may be overlooked, and those occult metastases may play critical roles in early-term cancer relapse after surgery. To identify hepatic micrometastases not detected by conventional methods, we employed indocyanine green (ICG) fluorescence imaging in real time during hepatobiliary and pancreatic cancer surgery. ***Patients/Methods:*** In this study, 125 consecutive patients were examined. Out of 125 patients, 99 had pancreatobiliary cancer and no evident hepatic tumors were apparent on clinical imaging, and 26 had colorectal cancer with overt hepatic metastases which were scheduled for excision. ICG was injected intravenously the day before surgery, and the liver was observed using a near-infrared camera system with laparotomy. The abnormal hepatic fluorescent foci were biopsied. Frozen tissue sections were examined histologically. ***Results:*** No adverse events related to the examination were evident. Hepatic micrometastases were confirmed in 17 patients (14%): 13 with pancreatobiliary cancer and 4 with colorectal cancer (in addition to their preoperatively overt metastases). The pancreatobiliary cancer patients with hepatic micrometastases were judged as having unresectable disease and underwent only palliative surgery. In the 4 patients with hepatic micrometastases from colorectal cancer, resection was intended to eradicate all of the metastases. Regardless of cancer origin, the patients with hepatic micrometastases received adjuvant systemic chemotherapy. Follow-up imaging studies within 12 months of surgery showed more frequent overt hepatic metastases in patients with micrometastases (13/14: 93%) than in those without (12/100: 12%; $p = 0.000$). ***Conclusions:*** ICG fluorescence imaging is useful for detection of hepatic micrometastases from digestive cancers and contributes to precise cancer staging. Hepatic micrometastases detected by this method had adverse clinical impacts which herald early-term hepatic relapse after surgery.

Hepatic metastases from digestive tract cancers rarely require radical resection because they are regarded as results of systemic cancer spread. Pancreatobiliary cancer patients with hepatic metastasis usually have extremely poor prognoses. These patients should be treated with systemic therapy, even if the metastases seem to be eradicable [1–3]. Hepatic metastasectomy may contribute to better prognoses exceptionally in colorectal cancer patients; however, hepatic relapse may occur if the metastases are not excised completely [4, 5]. Either way, precise assessment of hepatic metastasis plays a pivotal role in the treatment of patients with digestive tract cancers.

ICG fluorescence imaging is a system for clinical evaluation of real-time blood flow, lymphatic flow or biliary flow [6, 7]. In 2009, Ishizawa et al. [8] reported that this system could visualize hepatic tumors with high sensitivity. Inspired by their findings, we applied ICG fluorescence imaging to intraoperative examination of patients with hepatobiliary and pancreatic cancers. We sought to identify occult hepatic micrometastases that were not apparent on conventional imaging [9]. In this chapter, we describe our procedure and results, and discuss the feasibility and clinical impact of ICG fluorescence imaging-assisted detection of hepatic micrometastases.

Methods

Patients

From July 2009 to June 2012, 125 consecutive patients were examined using ICG fluorescence imaging. Within this group, there were 99 patients who underwent surgical laparotomy for pancreatobiliary cancer with no apparent hepatic tumor and 26 patients with colorectal cancer in who gross overt hepatic metastases had been identified. Preoperative clinical images had revealed 1–4 (median: 2) overt hepatic tumors in colorectal cancer patients with hepatic metastases.

Preparation

On the day before the surgery, 50 mg of ICG diluted with distilled water to a concentration of 2.5 mg/ml was intravenously injected. Patients with obstructive jaundice are not good candidates for this examination because diffuse bile stagnation causes nonspecific fluorescence in the entire liver. Therefore, biliary decompression was performed before the injection. ICG causes allergic reaction on rare occasions (0.17%). Therefore, prior to the procedure, patients were informed about the aim, procedure and complications of this examination before consent was obtained.

Detection of Hepatic Micrometastases

After laparotomy, intraoperative examinations with gross inspection and ultrasonography were performed for detecting hepatic disease. Subsequently, the Photodynamic Eye (PDE; Hamamatsu Photonics, Hamamatsu, Japan) fluorescence camera system was used with the surgical lights turned off. The camera head was positioned about 15 cm above the liver surface and the image was displayed on a television monitor. In order to examine the whole liver in detail, the liver was mobilized with dissecting round and falciform ligaments (fig. 1).

On PDE observation, lesions with biliary retention exhibit fluorescence. Thus, extra biliary tracts were used as inner positive controls. In patients with overt metastases from colorectal cancer, the tumors were also examined regardless of whether they fluoresced. In addition to inner fluorescence controls, benign hepatic lesions (i.e. biliary cysts, focal biliary retention or biliary hamartoma) fluoresced. Most of the benign fluorescence was easily recognized by gross inspection and palpation, but intraoperative histological examination was sometimes needed to distinguish benign lesions from hepatic micrometastases [9].

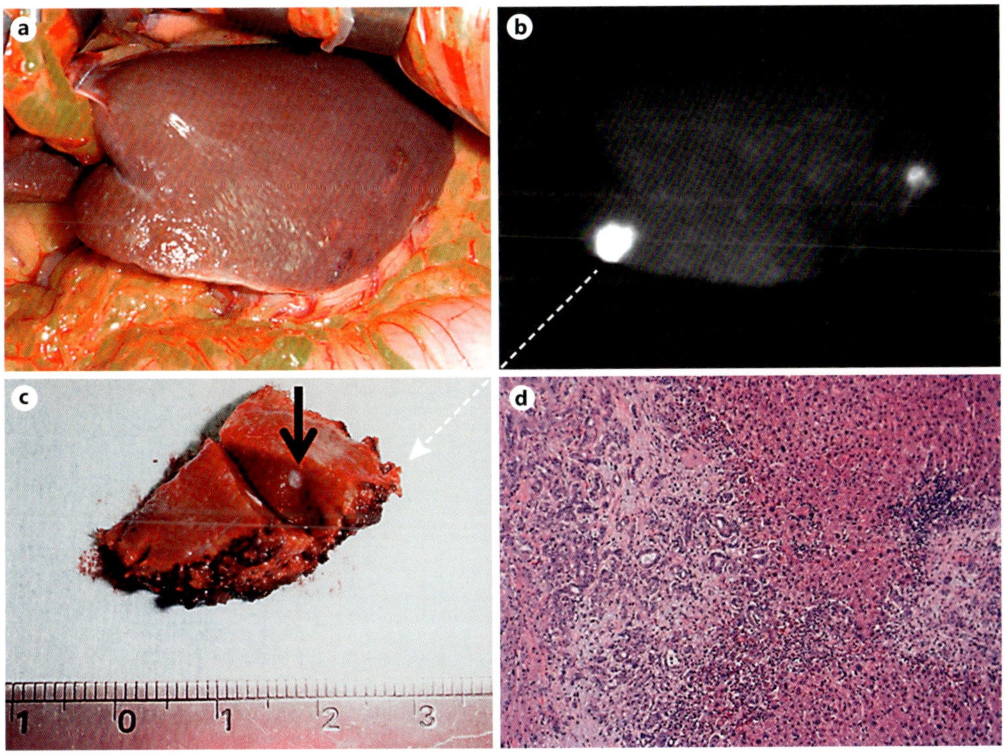

Fig. 1. a Representative case of hepatic micrometastases from pancreatic cancer. Although hepatic tumors were not evident upon gross inspection, 2 fluorescent spots were identified in the lateral segment by ICG fluorescence imaging and biopsied (white arrow) (**b**), a hepatic tumor <2 mm in diameter was observed below the fluorescence (black arrow) (**c**) and metastatic adenocarcinoma was histologically identified (**d**).

Fluorescent foci which could not be identified as benign or malignant by gross inspection were dissected and examined using frozen section histology (fig. 1). Multiple sections were made for histological examination because micrometastases were not always just on the fluorescent areas and the metastases might be so small that cut sections displace the lesions. If histological examination did not identify micrometastases in the cut sample, florescence results were recorded as 'false-positive florescence'.

Treatment Principles

When hepatic micrometastases were confirmed by ICG fluorescence imaging, surgical treatment and chemotherapies were planned as follows. In patients with pancreatobiliary cancer, palliative surgery was performed even if the micrometastases and primary cancer seemed to be resectable. These patients subsequently received systemic chemotherapy with gemcitabine [9, 10]. In patients with liver metastases from colorectal cancer, the resection line was planned to eradicate all of the overt and micrometastases. Patients received adjuvant chemotherapies using 5-fluorouracil and oxaliplatin (mFOLFOX6 regimen), or leucovorin calcium (calcium folinate), 5-fluorouracil and irinotecan (FOLFIRI regimen) [11, 12]. All 125 patients received follow-up CT or MRI 6 and 12 months after surgery to examine hepatic relapse.

Table 1. Hepatic micrometastases identified by ICG fluorescence imaging

Disease	Histologically confirmed hepatic micrometastases		
	positive[b]	false-positive[c]	negative[d]
Pancreatic cancer	11	5	50
Biliary tract cancer	2	2	29
Colorectal cancer[a]	4	0	21

[a] Surgically treated colorectal cancer patients with previous excision plans for overt hepatic metastases.
[b] Micrometastases were identified after biopsy of the fluorescent lesion.
[c] Although abnormal hepatic fluorescence was observed; micrometastases were not confirmed.
[d] Abnormal hepatic fluorescence was not observed.

Results

In the 125 patients examined, no adverse events related to the ICG injection or PDE were detected. Occult hepatic micrometastases were identified in 17 patients (14%) by fluorescence imaging and frozen section histology (table 1). False-positive florescence occurred in 7 patients (6%). Follow-up CT or MRI studies within 12 months after surgery showed that overt hepatic metastases appeared more frequently (13/14: 93%) in patients with histologically confirmed micrometastases than in those without (12/100: 12%; $p = 0.000$; Fisher's exact test).

Hepatic Micrometastases from Pancreatobiliary Cancer
Hepatic micrometastases were examined in 66 patients with pancreatic cancer and 33 patients with biliary tract cancer. During laparotomy, small nodules less than 3 mm were found on the hepatic surface and were suspected to be micrometastases in 3 patients. In the other 96 patients, hepatic tumor was not apparent by gross inspection or intraoperative ultrasonography. The ICG-infrared camera system showed abnormal hepatic fluorescence in 20 patients. The abnormal fluorescence in these patients ranged from small spots of less than 1.5 mm in diameter to wedge shaped segments of more than 3 cm^2. Among the 20 patients, hepatic micrometastases were histologically identified in biopsied tissue from 13 patients (11 had pancreatic cancer and 2 had biliary tract cancer) including the 3 patients in who micrometastases were suspected macroscopically. False-positive fluorescence occurred in 7 patients. These patients were treated as cases without hepatic metastases and subsequently underwent radical resection (4 patients) or palliative surgery (3 patients) in reference to their surgical staging.

On follow-up CT within 12 months after surgery, overt metastases were detected in 9 of the 10 patients (90%) with hepatic micrometastases. The hepatic tumors detected upon follow-up were larger in size and more numerous than those found at the time of surgery. In contrast, in 81 patients without micrometastases, hepatic tumors occurred in only 7 patients (9%). Of these 7 patients, 4 had false-positive fluorescence

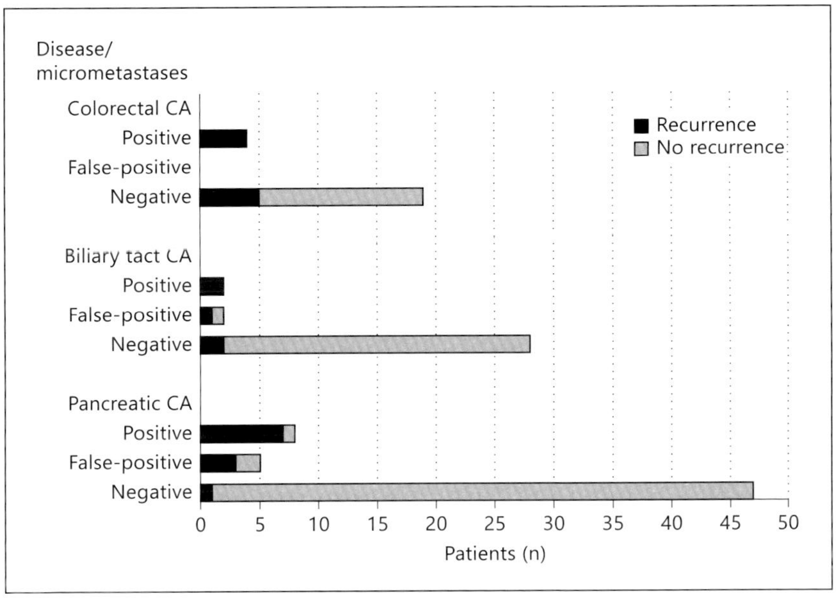

Fig. 2. Manifestation of overt hepatic metastases within 12 months after surgery. Patients were divided into 3 groups: those with positive fluorescence and histologically confirmed hepatic micrometastases, those with false-positive fluorescence (without confirmed micrometastases) and those with negative fluorescence. Patients with short-term follow-up periods (<12 months after surgery) were not included in the chart. CA = Cancer.

(fig. 2). The positive predictive value of the abnormal hepatic fluorescence for hepatic relapse within 12 months after surgery was 81% (13/16), independent of histological confirmation, and the negative predictive value was 95% (4/75).

Hepatic Micrometastases from Colorectal Cancer

Among 26 patients examined, preoperatively identified main hepatic tumors were identified as distinct fluorescence by PDE observation in 25 patients. Other than those evident tumors, abnormal fluorescent spots of less than 5 mm in diameter were found in 4 patients on the hepatic surface, although tumors were not evident upon gross inspection, and histological examination confirmed micrometastases in the hepatic parenchyma just below the fluorescence. Patients had 2–6 hepatic micrometastases. These lesions were located around the gross metastases in 2 patients and scattered in distant hepatic sectors in another 2 patients.

Considered as cases of tumor distribution, 3 patients with hepatic micrometastases underwent radical resection with the intention to excise all lesions. One patient was judged as having unresectable lesions because the metastases had dispersed throughout the entire liver. Twelve-month follow-up examinations showed that hepatic relapse occurred in all patients, including the patients who underwent radical resection (100%). In the patients without hepatic micrometastases, overt hepatic metastases were detected in 5 patients (5/19, 26%; fig. 2).

Discussion

Assessment of liver tumors has mainly depended on radiological modalities because endoscopic approaches for liver are difficult to perform, unlike other organs of the alimentally system. Recent developments in clinical imaging have made it possible to detect haptic tumors of less than 1 cm in diameter. However, extremely small tumors may be overlooked, even by advanced clinical imaging, and occult tumors may play critical roles in early-term cancer relapse after surgery [13–16]. As reported earlier, ICG fluorescence imaging enables practitioners to identify hepatic tumors with high sensitivity [8, 9]. Indeed, we identified hepatic micrometastases that were not detected by conventional imaging modalities in 14% of patients with pancreatobiliary and colorectal cancers. Some of these hepatic micrometastases might have been detectable through persistent palpation or very careful intraoperative ultrasonography. However, most of them may not been detected without the objective guide of fluorescence.

We analyzed final cancer staging and planned treatment strategies for each case in reference to results of the ICG fluorescence study. The outcomes of our patients demonstrated considerable clinical impacts. In pancreatobiliary cancer, rapid hepatic recurrence often manifests even after radical surgery. The prognosis of these cases are often extremely poor [14–16]. We encountered 16 patients with pancreatobiliary cancer in whom hepatic relapse occurred within 12 months after surgery. Eighty percent of these patients had abnormal findings by ICG fluorescence examination. Furthermore, histology confirmed that hepatic micrometastases led to overt tumors with high frequency (90%). These results suggest that the most of the early hepatic relapses in pancreatobiliary cancer were not metachronous, but instead simultaneous metastases which could not be identified due to their miniscule sizes at the time of surgery. Hepatic micrometastases may be evidence of widespread hepatic disease. Therefore, pancreatobiliary cancer patients with hepatic micrometastases should be treated in the same manner as those with evident metastases. We suggest that these patients do not warrant radical resection. On the other hand, patients without hepatic abnormal fluorescent were at low risk for liver deterioration after surgery. Thus, these patients may be good candidates for radical resection.

It is still unclear why hepatic metastases fluoresce by ICG-infrared imaging. The cause of a false-positive fluorescence signal is also unknown. As fluorescing hepatic areas were considerably larger than the actual tumor volume and their locations did not always correspond to those of the actual tumors, hepatic micrometastases did not seem to fluoresce themselves. We hypothesized that cancer tissue at the portal triad caused local biliary stasis, and the stagnant bile fluoresced under infrared illumination [9]. Although the penetration depth of infrared light in human tissue is limited, fluorescence on the hepatic surface may reflect metastatic foci in deep hepatic section, as it were, 'screen' [17]. Some of the false-positive cases may have micrometastases outside the collected sections. Alternatively, even if the collected samples contained cancerous tissue, histological studies may have missed the micrometastases because of their extremely small sizes. False-positive fluorescence should be explored in further basic science and clinical studies. Patients with false-positive fluorescence should be provisionally registered and hepatic recurrence should be monitored after surgery. We nevertheless argue that detection of hepatic micrometastases by ICG fluorescence imaging will contribute to precise cancer staging. Appropriate treatment strategies, based on the findings, may result in a decrease of early hepatic relapse after surgery for pancreatobiliary cancers.

In contrast to our original expectations, we obtained similar results in patients with colorectal cancer as in those with pancreatobiliary cancers. We intended to eradicate hepatic metastases from colorectal cancer patients including frank tumors and micrometastases. However, hepatic recurrence occurred in all patients with hepatic micrometastases. Previously, we published a histochemical study on resected liver specimens, with the aim of detecting hepatic micrometastases in patients with colorectal cancer. In that study, microlesions around the gross tumor were found immunohistochemically in 70% of the cases. These lesions were associated with hepatic recurrence after surgery [5]. These results are largely consistent with our present findings. Detection of micrometastases revealed a larger number and wider distribution of hepatic metastases. It is controversial as to whether the number of hepatic metastases may affect the probabilities of cancer relapse after hepatectomy; however, it would be difficult to achieve curative resection for widespread hepatic disease [18]. Additional occult micrometastases might be present in the preserved liver, despite the use of ICG fluorescence imaging. Our data suggest that hepatic micrometastases have an adverse clinical impact, not only in pancreatobiliary cancer but also in colorectal cancer. We also suggest that because conventional systemic chemotherapies could not prevent hepatic deterioration, other therapeutic approaches (i.e. liver perfusion chemotherapy, radiation therapy) are needed for patients with hepatic micrometastases regardless of cancer type [19–22].

Conclusions

Detection of hepatic micrometastases with ICG fluorescence imaging provides useful information for precise cancer staging. Although several limitations exist (i.e. penetration limits of infrared light, false-positive fluorescence), this examination can be performed with ease and a low risk of complications. Application of this method with laparoscopic or nonsurgical approaches from outside the body holds promise for a more convenient and less invasive method of examination [23]. Hepatic micrometastases detected through this examination predict early-term hepatic relapse after surgery. Additional studies that clarify the pathological and biological features of hepatic micrometastases are needed in order to overcome this disease.

References

1 Shukla PJ, Neve R, Barreto SG, et al: Pancreatic resection for M1 pancreatic ductal adenocarcinoma. Ann Surg Oncol 2007;14:118–127.

2 Seelig S, Burkert B, Chromik A, Tannapfel A, Uhl W, Seelig M: Pancreatic resections for advanced M1-pancreatic carcinoma: the value of synchronous metastasectomy. HPB Surg 2010;2010:579672.

3 Gleisner AL, Assumpcao L, Cameron J, et al: Is resection of periampullary or pancreatic adenocarcinoma with synchronous hepatic metastasis justified? Cancer 2007;110:2484–2492.

4 Jamison R, Donohue J, Nagorney D, et al: Hepatic resection for metastatic cancer results in cure for some patients. Arch Surg 1997;132:505–511.

5 Yokoyama N, Shirai Y, Ajioka Y, Nagakura S, Suda T, Hatakeyama H: Immunohistochemically detected hepatic micrometastases predict a high risk of intrahepatic recurrence after resection of colorectal carcinoma liver metastases. Cancer 2002;94:1642–1647.

6 Taggart DP, Choudhary B, Anastasiadis K, Abu-Omer Y, Balacumaraswami L, Pigott D: Preliminary experience with a novel intraoperative fluorescence imaging technique to evaluate the patency of bypass grafts in total arterial revascularization. Ann Thorac Surg 2003;75:870–873.

7 Ishizawa T, Bandai Y, Kokudo N: Fluorescent cholangiography using indocyanine green for laparoscopic cholecystectomy: an initial experience. Arch Surg 2009;144:381–382.

8 Ishizawa T, Fukushima N, Shibahara J, et al: Real-time identification of liver cancers by using indocyanine green fluorescent imaging. Cancer 2009;115:2491–2504.

9 Yokoyama N, Otani T, Hashidate H, et al: Real-time detection of hepatic micrometastases from pancreatic cancer by intraoperative fluorescence imaging: preliminary results of a prospective study. Cancer 2012;118:2813–2819.

10 Burris HA 3rd, Moore MJ, Andersen J, et al: Improvements in survival and clinical benefit with gemcitabine as first-line therapy for patients with advanced pancreas cancer: a randomized trial. J Clin Oncol 1997;15:2403–2413.

11 Cheeseman S, Joel S, Chester J, et al: A 'modified de Gramont' regimen of fluorouracil, alone and with oxaliplatin, for advanced colorectal cancer. Br J Cancer 2002;87:393–399.

12 Douillard JY, Cunningham D, Roth AD, et al: Irinotecan combined with fluorouracil compared with fluorouracil alone as first-line treatment for metastatic colorectal cancer: a multicentre randomised trial. Lancet 2000;355:1041–1047.

13 Zamboni GA, Kruskal JB, Vollmer CM, Baptista J, Callery MP, Raptopoulos VD: Pancreatic adenocarcinoma: value of multidetector CT angiography in preoperative evaluation. Radiology 2007;245:770–778.

14 Amikura K, Kobari M, Matsuno S: The time of occurrence of liver metastasis in carcinoma of the pancreas. Int J Pancreatol 1995;17:139–146.

15 Griffin JF, Smalley SR, Jewell W, et al: Patterns of failure after curative resection of pancreatic carcinoma. Cancer 1990;66:56–61.

16 Takao S, Shinchi H, Uchikura K, Kubo M, Aikou T: Liver metastases after curative resection in patients with distal bile duct cancer. Br J Surg 1999;86:327–331.

17 Mitsuhashi N, Kimura F, Shimizu H, et al: Usefulness of intraoperative fluorescence imaging to evaluate local anatomy in hepatobiliary surgery. J Hepatobiliary Pancreat Surg 2008;15:508–514.

18 Saiura A, Yamamoto J, Hasegawa K, et al: Liver resection for multiple colorectal liver metastases with surgery up-front approach: bi-institutional analysis of 736 consecutive cases. World J Surg 2012;36:2171–2178.

19 Hishinuma S, Ogata Y, Tomikawa M, et al: Prophylactic hepatic irradiation following curative resection of pancreatic cancer. J Hepatobiliary Pancreat Surg 2005;12:235–242.

20 Morak M, van der Gaast A, Incrocci L, et al: Adjuvant intra-arterial chemotherapy and radiotherapy versus surgery alone in resectable pancreatic and periampullary cancer: a prospective randomized controlled trial. Ann Surg 2008;248:1031–1041.

21 Kurosaki I, Kawachi Y, Nihei K, et al: Liver perfusion chemotherapy with 5-fluorouracil followed by systemic gemcitabine administration for resected pancreatic cancer: preliminary results of a prospective phase 2 study. Pancreas 2009;38:161–167.

22 Elaraj D, Alexander H: Current role of hepatic artery infusion and isolated liver perfusion for the treatment of colorectal cancer liver metastases. Cancer J 2004;10:128–138.

23 Miyashiro I, Kishi K, Yano M, et al: Laparoscopic detection of sentinel node in gastric cancer by indocyanine green imaging. Surg Endosc 2011;25:1672–1676.

Naoyuki Yokoyama, MD, PhD
Department of Digestive Surgery, Niigata City General Hospital
463-7 Shumoku, Chuo-ku
Niigata City, 950-1197 (Japan)
E-Mail yokonao@hosp.niigata.niigata.jp

Kokudo N, Ishizawa T (eds): Fluorescent Imaging: Treatment of Hepatobiliary and Pancreatic Diseases.
Front Gastrointest Res. Basel, Karger, 2013, vol 31, pp 33–41 (DOI: 10.1159/000348602)

Application of Fluorescence Imaging to Hepatopancreatobiliary Surgery

Merlijn Hutteman · Floris P.R. Verbeek · Alexander L. Vahrmeijer

Department of Surgery, Leiden University Medical Center, Leiden, The Netherlands

Abstract

Over the last century, improved imaging methods and surgical techniques have modernized hepatopancreatobiliary (HPB) surgery. However, visual inspection, palpation and intraoperative ultrasound are the primary methods of determining what structures need to be resected during surgery. Using these methods, accurate identification of structures can be challenging, especially in laparoscopic HPB surgery, where palpation is not possible. This can result in irradical resections and iatrogenic damage to vital structures. Intraoperative imaging using near-infrared (NIR) fluorescence can be used for real-time assessment of both anatomy and function. In this chapter, the current status of (clinical) applications of NIR fluorescence imaging using indocyanine green during HPB surgery is evaluated. NIR fluorescence imaging combines the use of NIR fluorescent contrast agents and specially designed imaging systems which are capable of detecting these contrast agents during surgery. In comparison with visible light, NIR fluorescent light can penetrate living tissue several millimeters deeper, providing improved detectability. In HPB surgery, intraoperative NIR fluorescence has been evaluated for tumor imaging in the liver and pancreas, and real-time imaging of the biliary tree. In these applications, NIR fluorescence imaging has been shown to be a promising new technique that may improve surgical accuracy and lower complications in the future.

Over the last century great improvements have been made in the field of hepatopancreatobiliary (HPB) surgery. Due to improved imaging techniques, more effective chemotherapy regimens and better, more aggressive surgical strategies, the survival after HPB surgery has strongly increased. Imaging technologies such as ultrasonography, computed tomography, magnetic resonance imaging, single-photon emission computed tomography and positron emission tomography are widely used for preoperative planning in HPB surgery [1]. Translation of preoperative images to the intraoperative setting remains a major challenge. Of the many imaging methods available, only ultrasound and fluoroscopy can be used in real time during surgery [1, 2]. Therefore, during HPB surgery, the surgeon still mainly has to rely on visual inspection and palpation to discriminate between structures that need to be resected (e.g. tumors, lymph nodes) and structures that need to be spared (e.g. bile ducts). As a result, irradical oncologic resections and iatrogenic surgical trauma are still major issues in HPB surgery.

Intraoperative imaging using near-infrared (NIR) fluorescence is a relatively new technique that can be used to visualize tumor tissue and vital anatomical structures. By using the physiological clearance of exogenous contrast agents, functional information as well as anatomical information can be acquired, such as for the liver and biliary tree. These characteristics make NIR fluorescence imaging a suitable imaging modality for intraoperative use in HPB surgery.

In this chapter, we describe the current status and clinical application of NIR fluorescence imaging for HPB surgery and future outlook.

Near-Infrared Fluorescence Imaging

NIR fluorescent light has several advantageous properties for intraoperative imaging. The wavelength of NIR light is between 700 and 900 nm, which is invisible to the human eye, and therefore does not alter the look of the surgical field. At this wavelength, light has relatively low tissue absorbance, resulting in high tissue penetration (up to 5 mm) and low autofluorescence. Neither ionizing radiation nor direct tissue contact is employed in NIR fluorescence imaging, making it an inherently safe technique. Images can be acquired within a few milliseconds to allow the surgeon to operate under real-time image guidance. The introduction of minimally invasive techniques has increased the need for additional intraoperative imaging modalities. For example, NIR fluorescence imaging has been used during robot-assisted laparoscopic surgery to optimize sentinel lymph node dissection [3].

Many imaging systems have been developed for intraoperative use, for both open and minimally invasive procedures. Several of these systems are commercially available. Descriptions of some of these systems are provided by Gioux et al. [4]. Optimized imaging systems have the ability to provide a real-time overlay of the NIR fluorescence signal with visible color images. This demonstrates the NIR fluorescence signal in relation to the surgical anatomy, enabling true image guidance.

Besides intraoperative imaging systems, for NIR fluorescence image-guided surgery, an NIR fluorescent contrast agent is also needed to visualize specific structures that need to be resected (e.g. tumor tissue) or should be spared (e.g. bile ducts). Indocyanine green (ICG) is currently the only NIR fluorophore that is registered with the Food and Drug Administration (FDA) and the European Medicines Agency (EMA) for clinical application, albeit for other indications. ICG has been used since the 1950s to measure cardiac output, hepatic function and retinal perfusion. The absorbance of ICG is around 800 nm and complications following administration are rare, making it a safe contrast agent. Most studies report ICG doses between 1 and 10 mg for intraoperative imaging applications, but intravenous injection up to 25 mg has been reported to be safe. After intravenous injection, ICG is cleared rapidly by the liver and almost completely excreted into the bile.

Methylene blue is also currently applicable for clinical use and at correct concentrations has fluorescent properties. However, its emission peak is around 700 nm, which is less optimal due to higher tissue absorbance and higher autofluorescence. Its use for HPB surgery is beyond the scope of the current chapter, but is reviewed in [5].

ICG cannot be conjugated to specific ligands due to its chemical structure, making it a nonspecific NIR contrast agent. Novel NIR fluorescent probes are being developed to permit targeted imaging, as recently reviewed by Luo et al. [6].

The various applications of intraoperative NIR fluorescence imaging using ICG are discussed in the following sections of this chapter.

Bile Imaging

Bile Duct Imaging

Common bile duct (CBD) injury is a rare but severe complication during (laparoscopic) cholecystectomy with a postoperative mortality of 11% [7]. In studies, intraoperative cholangiography has been shown to reduce the risk of CBD injury from 0.58 to 0.39% [7]. However, the advantage of routine cholangiography has been doubted. Intraoperative cholangiography is time consuming and the introduction of a catheter into the CBD can induce leakage. Laparoscopic ultrasonography is a less invasive and safe method to identify stones in the CBD and anatomical abnormalities, but it is not widely used.

The use of NIR fluorescence imaging is a safe alternative to image biliary anatomy and function during hepatobiliary surgery. Most studies exploit the biliary excretion of ICG after intravenous injection of ICG to perform NIR fluorescence cholangiography. Some studies also employed retrograde injection of an NIR fluorophore in the CBD. However, as with fluoroscopic cholangiography, this can result in iatrogenic damage.

In most studies that used ICG for intravenous injection, ICG was injected 30 min prior to surgery, and most studies used a dose of 2.5 mg (with the exception of one study that reported the use of 12.5 mg ICG [8]). Using fluorescence cholangiography during laparoscopic cholecystectomy, Aoki et al. [8] showed identification of the CBD and cystic duct in 10 of 14 patients. The authors stated that unsuccessful identification of the bile ducts was caused by obesity. In the unsuccessfully imaged patients, fatty tissue around the bile ducts hampered visualization.

To optimize dose and analyze biodistribution over time, Hutteman et al. [9] visualized the CBD and cholangiojejunostomy during open pancreaticoduodenectomy after intravenous injection of ICG in 8 patients (fig 1). Between 10 and 90 min after administration of 5 and 10 mg of ICG, the CBD could clearly be identified by NIR fluorescence imaging in all patients. No difference was observed between the 5-mg

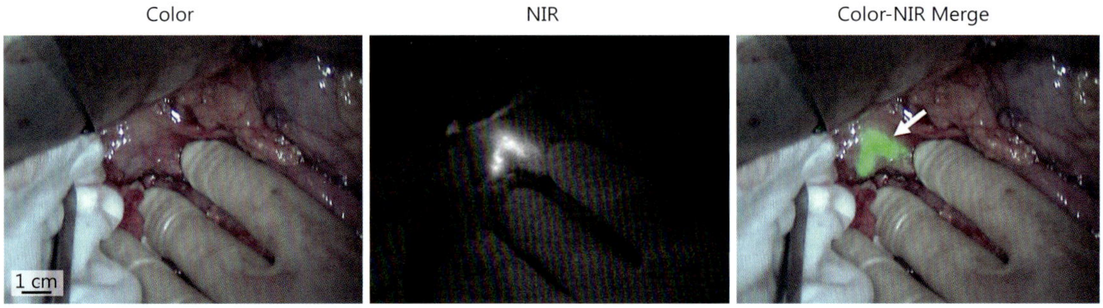

Fig. 1. NIR fluorescence imaging of the bile duct during liver surgery. Color image (left panel), NIR fluorescence (middle panel) and a color-NIR overlay (right panel) of intraoperative imaging of the CBD in a patient who underwent a cholecystectomy during previous surgery, 30 min after administration of 5 mg of ICG. A clear contrast is shown between the CBD (arrow) and surrounding tissue.

and 10-mg groups. The highest signal-to-background ratios were found between 30 and 90 min postinjection.

In conclusion, for intraoperative NIR fluorescence cholangiography, dose and timing of contrast agent administration are important factors. From the currently available clinical literature, the most optimal parameters to perform clinical NIR fluorescence bile duct imaging appear to be the administration of 2.5 mg of ICG approximately 30 min prior to surgery.

Bile Leakage Imaging

Bile leakage is one of the most feared complications after HPB surgery and its occurrence is strongly related to perioperative mortality [10]. Detection of a bile leak at an early stage could potentially prevent severe complications, such as liver failure. Two clinical studies have described the use of NIR fluorescence for bile leakage identification after hepatic resection [11, 12]. ICG was injected intrabiliarily after hepatic resection using a transcystic catheter. The CBD was clamped distal to the cystic duct and NIR fluorescence imaging was performed. In 102 patients undergoing hepatic resection, 5 patients developed postoperative bile leakage in the control group versus no patients in the group in which NIR fluorescence was used ($p = 0.019$) [11]. This demonstrates the clinical applicability of NIR fluorescence imaging for intraoperative detection of bile leakage and suggests positive effects on patient outcome.

Tumor Imaging

Liver Cancer and Colorectal Metastases

An estimated 748,300 new cases and 695,900 cancer deaths related to liver cancer were reported worldwide in 2008. Colorectal cancer is the second cause of cancer death

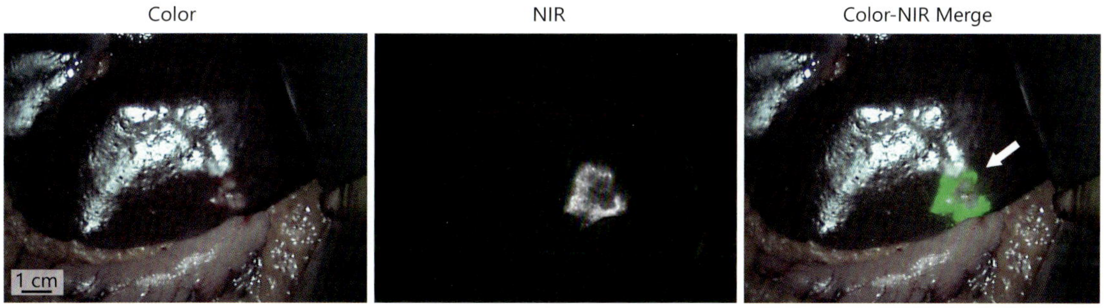

Fig. 2. NIR fluorescence imaging of colorectal liver metastases. A CLM (arrow) is clearly identified by a NIR fluorescent rim around the tumor in vivo, 24 h after injection of 10 mg of ICG. Normal liver tissue shows minimal retention of ICG.

worldwide and the survival of colorectal carcinoma patients depends a great deal on the occurrence of distant metastases, most frequently localized in the liver. Advanced surgical techniques, preoperative imaging and (neoadjuvant) chemotherapy regiments have led to an increased proportion of patients eligible for resection of liver tumors. During resection of liver tumors, visual inspection, palpation and intraoperative ultrasound are commonly used to determine the extent of the disease. However, reported recurrence rates of colorectal liver metastases (CLM) vary between 11 and 37.5%, of which 65–85% occur within 2 years following surgery [13, 14]. The high recurrence rate could possibly be explained by the presence of small malignant lesions that are missed intraoperatively by the currently used detection methods.

NIR fluorescence imaging using ICG could potentially aid the intraoperative identification of primary liver tumors and CLM. As it is impossible to palpate the liver surface during laparoscopic surgery, NIR fluorescence imaging could have particular added value during minimally invasive liver surgery. In hepatocellular carcinoma patients, ICG has been shown to passively accumulate in the tumor (fig. 2). In CLM patients, ICG has been shown to accumulate as a rim around the tumor. In both groups, ICG was intravenously administered 1–14 days before surgery [15]. As accumulation of ICG in liver tumors is based on pharmacokinetic clearance, it is probably influenced by liver perfusion, ICG uptake and clearance by the liver and biliary drainage.

Several clinical studies describe the use of NIR fluorescence imaging to visualize hepatocellular carcinoma and CLM. A detailed description of the application of NIR fluorescence imaging for intraoperative hepatocellular carcinoma detection can be found in Ishizawa and Kokudo [this vol., 1–9]. A number of clinical studies have described the use of ICG for visualization of CLM, and are described in detail in Lim and Vibert [this vol., 18–24].

Van der Vorst et al. [16] (Cancer, accepted for publication) examined the use of NIR fluorescence imaging for the intraoperative detection of CLM metastases using ICG in 40 consecutive patients and observed similar results. Additionally, ICG dosing and timing were optimized. Importantly, in this study, in 5 of 40 patients (12.5%, 95% CI: 5.0–26.6), additional small and superficially located lesions were detected using NIR fluorescence, and were otherwise undetectable by preoperative computed tomography, intraoperative ultrasound, visualization and palpation. Moreover, this study showed that NIR fluorescence imaging appears capable of differentiating between benign and malignant tumors. In 13 patients, benign liver lesions were identified intraoperatively. These lesions could be clearly differentiated from malignant lesions due to the lack of NIR fluorescent signal in the lesion and the lack of a fluorescent rim around them.

The potential of this technique to detect small hepatic metastases was studied in pancreatic cancer patients. Forty-nine patients with pancreatic cancer who were undergoing surgical resection with curative intent were included. In these patients, no hepatic tumors were identified using preoperative imaging or intraoperatively by inspection or ultrasonography. After injection of 25 mg of ICG [17], NIR fluorescence imaging detected abnormal lesions in the liver in 13 patients. In 8 out of 13 lesions, micrometastases were found. This demonstrates that NIR fluorescence imaging can be of added value to detect hepatic metastases of pancreatic cancer that were otherwise undetected. This could help surgeons select patients for either curative or palliative treatment.

NIR fluorescence imaging after preoperative ICG administration was also used to visualize cholestatic liver parenchyma intraoperatively [18]. In a pilot study, 2 patients with intrahepatic cholangiocarcinoma and 1 patient with CLM metastases and a suspected bile duct thrombus were imaged. Using NIR fluorescence imaging, the cholestatic regions on the surface of the liver caused by bile duct tumor invasion or thrombi could be detected in all 3 patients [18].

In conclusion, several studies have shown that intraoperative NIR fluorescence imaging using ICG is feasible for liver tumor detection and segmental demarcation. The major hurdle for this technique is the limited detectability of NIR fluorescence at deeper localized tissue, which is currently limited at around 5 mm. Current research is focused on optimizing techniques to improve detection at higher depths. Furthermore, NIR fluorescence imaging could be of added value for the detection of small superficial lesions

Pancreatic Cancer

Pancreatic adenocarcinoma is the fourth leading cause of cancer death in Western countries. The overall 5-year survival rate is less than 5% and has not substantially improved over the past 30 years. The main prognostic factor for pancreatic cancer patients after curative intended resection is the occurrence of tumor-positive resection margins. Median survival rates after a microscopically complete (R0) resection for pancreatic adenocarcinoma are twice as high when compared to a R1 resection [19]. Irradical resections are reported in 34.7–42% of patients undergoing resection of pancreatic cancers [20–22]. Novel and optimized preoperative imaging methods have improved preoperative planning. However, similar to hepatic tumors, translation of these images and techniques to the intraoperative setting is still a challenge.

To date, only one clinical study has described attempts to visualize pancreatic tumors using NIR fluorescence imaging after ICG injection. Previous work has shown that passive accumulation due the enhanced permeability and retention effect can be used to identify solid tumors. Hutteman et al. [9] attempted to use this concept for pancreatic cancer imaging after ICG injection. However, the results were disappointing. After intravenous injection of ICG, intraoperative visualization of a pancreatic tumor was observed in only 1 of 8 patients. A possible explanation could be sought in lower perfusion of adenocarcinomas of the pancreas in comparison with healthy pancreatic tissue. This could decrease effective circulation of ICG in the tumor for a potential accumulation by an enhanced permeability and retention effect.

Hirono et al. [23] used NIR fluorescence imaging to analyze lymphatic drainage patterns in pancreatic cancer using local ICG injections. In 20 patients, ICG was injected into the pancreas head, and lymphatic flow could be visualized in all patients. This method can provide important insights into patterns of lymphatic metastases in pancreatic cancer.

Discussion

Image-guidance during HPB surgery by means of intraoperative NIR fluorescence imaging has been found to be useful in a variety of applications. It has been studied in intraoperative identification of tumors and vital structures. Applications of this technique include the identification and demarcation of HPB tumors, identification of pancreatic liver metastases, real-time cholangiography and bile leakage detection. By exploiting the hepatic clearance of ICG, it is also possible to acquire functional images of the liver and biliary system.

The availability of ICG for clinical application has allowed NIR fluorescence image-guided surgery to be introduced into clinical trials. However, to allow this technique to have a chance to become the standard of care for tumor imaging, tumor-targeted contrast agents will be essential. In the current literature, many preclinical studies have shown encouraging results using (experimental) tumor-specific probes. An important factor hampering the clinical implementation of these probes is the fact that each of these probes has to go through a separate expensive and time-consuming regulatory approval processes.

Another important factor for clinical acceptance of this technique will be the continued development of imaging systems, as a large proportion of currently used imaging systems are still in the experimental phase. Novel systems have shown improved image quality and resolution, better sensitivity and increased usability. In the last few years, the proportion of laparoscopic HPB procedures has steadily increased, making it of particular interest for the development and improvement of laparoscopic fluorescence imaging systems. With currently broadly employed planar imaging, quantification in optical imaging remains challenging and are influenced by varying tissue absorbance and probe concentration at the site that is imaged. One of the major limiting factors of NIR fluorescence imaging is its limited tissue penetration depth. Currently available studies report a penetration depth ranging from several millimeters to, at most, 1 cm. Current research on imaging system development is focused on new detection methods to improve signal quantification and detection of fluorescence signals located deeper within tissue, such as by means of time domain imaging and spatial frequency domain imaging [24, 25].

Besides optimization of NIR fluorescent contrast agents and imaging systems, large clinical trials will be essential to validate the use of NIR fluorescence imaging, and eventually to assess true patient benefit. Despite the very promising results already obtained, the next decade will show if NIR fluorescence imaging during HPB surgery delivers benefits to routine patient care.

References

1 Miura F, Takada T, Amano H, Yoshida M, Furui S, Takeshita K: Diagnosis of pancreatic cancer. HPB (Oxford) 2006;8:337–342.

2 Ezaki T, Stansby GP, Hobbs KE: Intraoperative ultrasonographic imaging in liver surgery: a review. HPB Surg 1990;3:1–4.

3 van der Poel HG, Buckle T, Brouwer OR, Valdes Olmos RA, van Leeuwen FW: Intraoperative laparoscopic fluorescence guidance to the sentinel lymph node in prostate cancer patients: clinical proof of concept of an integrated functional imaging approach using a multimodal tracer. Eur Urol 2011;60: 826–833.

4 Gioux S, Choi HS, Frangioni JV: Image-guided surgery using invisible near-infrared light: fundamentals of clinical translation. Mol Imaging 2010;9:237–255.

5 Verbeek FP, van der Vorst JR, Schaafsma BE, Hutteman M, Bonsing BA, van Leeuwen FW, Frangioni JV, van de Velde CJ, Swijnenburg RJ, Vahrmeijer AL: Image-guided hepatopancreatobiliary surgery using near-infrared fluorescent light. J Hepatobiliary Pancreat Sci 2012;19:626–637.

6 Luo S, Zhang E, Su Y, Cheng T, Shi C: A review of NIR dyes in cancer targeting and imaging. Biomaterials 2011;32:7127–7138.

7 Flum DR, Koepsell T, Heagerty P, Sinanan M, Dellinger EP: Common bile duct injury during laparoscopic cholecystectomy and the use of intraoperative cholangiography: adverse outcome or preventable error? Arch Surg 2001;136:1287–1292.

8 Aoki T, Murakami M, Yasuda D, Shimizu Y, Kusano T, Matsuda K, Niiya T, Kato H, Murai N, Otsuka K, Kusano M, Kato T: Intraoperative fluorescent imaging using indocyanine green for liver mapping and cholangiography. J Hepatobiliary Pancreat Surg 2009;17:590–594.

9 Hutteman M, van der Vorst JR, Mieog JS, Bonsing BA, Hartgrink HH, Kuppen PJ, Lowik CW, Frangioni JV, van de Velde CJ, Vahrmeijer AL: Near-infrared fluorescence imaging in patients undergoing pancreaticoduodenectomy. Eur Surg Res 2011;47: 90–97.

10 Yamashita Y, Hamatsu T, Rikimaru T, Tanaka S, Shirabe K, Shimada M, Sugimachi K: Bile leakage after hepatic resection. Ann Surg 2001;233:45–50.

11 Kaibori M, Ishizaki M, Matsui K, Hon KA: Intraoperative indocyanine green fluorescent imaging for prevention of bile leakage after hepatic resection. Surgery 2011;150:91–98.

12 Sakaguchi T, Suzuki A, Unno N, Morita Y, Oishi K, Fukumoto K, Inaba K, Suzuki M, Tanaka H, Sagara D, Suzuki S, Nakamura S, Konno H: Bile leak test by indocyanine green fluorescence images after hepatectomy. Am J Surg 2010;200:e19–e23.

13 Abdalla EK, Vauthey JN, Ellis LM, Ellis V, Pollock R, Broglio KR, Hess K, Curley SA: Recurrence and outcomes following hepatic resection, radiofrequency ablation, and combined resection/ablation for colorectal liver metastases. Ann Surg 2004;239:818–825.

14 Karanjia ND, Lordan JT, Fawcett WJ, Quiney N, Worthington TR: Survival and recurrence after neoadjuvant chemotherapy and liver resection for colorectal metastases: a ten year study. Eur J Surg Oncol 2009;35:838–843.
15 Ishizawa T, Fukushima N, Shibahara J, Masuda K, Tamura S, Aoki T, Hasegawa K, Beck Y, Fukayama M, Kokudo N: Real-time identification of liver cancers by using indocyanine green fluorescent imaging. Cancer 2009;115:2491–2504.
16 van der Vorst JR, Schaafsma BE, Hutteman M, Verbeek FP, Liefers GJ, Hartgrink HH, Smit VT, Lowik CW, van de velde CJ, Frangioni JV, Vahrmeijer AL: Near infrared fluorescence-Guided Resection of colorectal liver metastases. Cancer, accepted for publication.
17 Yokoyama N, Otani T, Hashidate H, Maeda C, Katada T, Sudo N, Manabe S, Ikeno Y, Toyoda A, Katayanagi N: Real-time detection of hepatic micrometastases from pancreatic cancer by intraoperative fluorescence imaging: preliminary results of a prospective study. Cancer 2011;118:2813–2819.
18 Harada N, Ishizawa T, Muraoka A, Ijichi M, Kusaka K, Shibasaki M, Yamamoto K, Hasegawa K, Bandai Y, Kokudo N: Fluorescence navigation hepatectomy by visualization of localized cholestasis from bile duct tumor infiltration. J Am Coll Surg 2010;210:e2–e6.
19 Garcea G, Dennison AR, Pattenden CJ, Neal CP, Sutton CD, Berry DP: Survival following curative resection for pancreatic ductal adenocarcinoma. A systematic review of the literature. JOP 2008;9:99–132.
20 Sommerville CA, Limongelli P, Pai M, Ahmad R, Stamp G, Habib NA, Williamson RC, Jiao LR: Survival analysis after pancreatic resection for ampullary and pancreatic head carcinoma: an analysis of clinicopathological factors. J Surg Oncol 2009;100: 651–656.
21 Kato K, Yamada S, Sugimoto H, Kanazumi N, Nomoto S, Takeda S, Kodera Y, Morita S, Nakao A: Prognostic factors for survival after extended pancreatectomy for pancreatic head cancer: influence of resection margin status on survival. Pancreas 2009; 38:605–612.
22 Winter JM, Cameron JL, Campbell KA, Arnold MA, Chang DC, Coleman J, Hodgin MB, Sauter PK, Hruban RH, Riall TS, Schulick RD, Choti MA, Lillemoe KD, Yeo CJ: 1423 pancreaticoduodenectomies for pancreatic cancer: a single-institution experience. J Gastrointest Surg 2006;10:1199–1210.
23 Hirono S, Tani M, Kawai M, Okada K, Miyazawa M, Shimizu A, Uchiyama K, Yamaue H: Identification of the lymphatic drainage pathways from the pancreatic head guided by indocyanine green fluorescence imaging during pancreaticoduodenectomy. Dig Surg 2012;29:132–139.
24 Kumar AT, Raymond SB, Bacskai BJ, Boas DA: Comparison of frequency-domain and time-domain fluorescence lifetime tomography. Opt Lett 2008;33: 470–472.
25 Mazhar A, Dell S, Cuccia DJ, Gioux S, Durkin AJ, Frangioni JV, Tromberg BJ: Wavelength optimization for rapid chromophore mapping using spatial frequency domain imaging. J Biomed Opt 2010;15: 061716.

Dr. Alexander L. Vahrmeijer
Albinusdreef 2
NL–2333 ZA Leiden (The Netherlands)
E-Mail a.l.vahrmeijer@lumc.nl

Kokudo N, Ishizawa T (eds): Fluorescent Imaging: Treatment of Hepatobiliary and Pancreatic Diseases.
Front Gastrointest Res. Basel, Karger, 2013, vol 31, pp 42–48 (DOI: 10.1159/000348604)

Applications of Indocyanine Green Fluorescence Imaging to Liver Transplantation

Yoshikuni Kawaguchi · Takeaki Ishizawa · Yasuhiko Sugawara · Norihiro Kokudo

Hepato-Biliary-Pancreatic Surgery Division, Department of Surgery, Graduate School of Medicine, The University of Tokyo, Tokyo, Japan

Abstract

Recently, fluorescence imaging using indocyanine green (ICG) has been applied to hepatobiliary surgery. Herein, the clinical applications of ICG fluorescence imaging in cases of liver transplantation are described. First, concomitant use of fluorescence cholangiography following intrabiliary injection of ICG by conventional radiographic cholangiography is useful for determination of the division point of the hepatic duct during donor surgery. Secondly, fluorescence angiography can be used to evaluate the hepatic blood flow after venous reconstruction in recipient surgery. Lastly, ICG fluorescence imaging enables simple and easy evaluation of the portal uptake function in hepatic regions with venous occlusion caused by the division of the major hepatic vein tributaries, information about which is helpful for surgeons to determine the operative indication and need for venous reconstruction, not only in liver transplantation, but also in major hepatic resections for malignancy.

Recently, a fluorescence imaging technique using indocyanine green (ICG) has been developed and clinically applied to intraoperative visualization of the bile ducts [1–3], liver cancers [4, 5] and hepatic segments to be resected [6, 7] in hepatobiliary surgery. Herein, the clinical applications of ICG fluorescence imaging in the field of liver transplantation are described.

In several countries facing a scarcity of deceased donors like Japan, living-donor liver transplantation (LDLT) remains the mainstay. As compared to deceased donor liver transplantation, more delicate and accurate surgical procedures are required for LDLT because the donor's safety needs priority, and in the case of recipient surgery, the diameter of the hepatic vessels and bile ducts to be anastomosed are thin. As in the case of liver resection for malignancy, ICG fluorescence imaging can also be utilized in LDLT procedures in order to identify the confluence of the left and right hepatic duct during surgery on the donor and to confirm the hepatic blood flow after vessel reconstruction during surgery in the recipient. Furthermore, the method for treating hepatic regions with venous occlusion caused by division of the major hepatic venous tributaries has recently become an important issue in LDLT as in liver resection since it has been unclear as to what extent the liver function in such veno-occlusive hepatic regions might decrease as a result of decreased or regurgitated portal flow. ICG fluorescence imaging may also be effective in estimating the function of a donor's future remnant liver with veno-occlusive regions and determining the indications for venous reconstruction made on the liver graft during recipient surgery [8, 9].

Clinical Application

Fluorescence Cholangiography during Donor Surgery

Administration of Indocyanine Green

Fluorescence cholangiography is performed by intrabiliary injection of ICG (0.025 mg/ml of Diagnogreen; Daiichi Sankyo Co., Tokyo, Japan) or by intravenous injection of ICG (1 ml, 2.5 mg) at least 15 min before the observation [10].

Identification of the Confluence of the Hepatic Ducts

The camera imaging head of the fluorescence imaging system is positioned about 20–50 cm above the hepatic hilum. The surgical light is turned off (only ceiling lights are kept on). ICG, diluted with radiographic contrast material (Omnipaque; Daiichi Sankyo Co.) to a concentration of 0.025 mg/ml, is injected into the bile duct through the transcystic tube. By diluting ICG with radiographic contrast material, fluorescence images of the confluence of the left and right hepatic ducts are visualized on the surrounding structures at the same time or just after radiographic cholangiography using a C-arm fluoroscopy machine to confirm the intrahepatic bile duct anatomy [3]. Fig. 1a shows a case of donor surgery for procurement of the right liver graft. In this case, a fluorescence imaging system which enables simultaneous visualization of ICG fluorescence on the color images (HyperEye Medical System, Mizuho Ikakogyo Co. Ltd., Tokyo, Japan) was used [3]. The right hepatic duct was divided by using fluorescence cholangiography in real time to determine the optimal point for the division, following confirmation of the intrahepatic bile duct anatomy by conventional radiographic cholangiography.

Clinical applications of fluorescence cholangiography have been reported by several authors [1–3, 10]. Among them, the major advantage of using the fluorescence imaging system described above is that it overlays fluorescence images on the background color images. This feature may make it easier for surgeons to understand the exact location of the fluorescing lesions, as compared to other commercially available

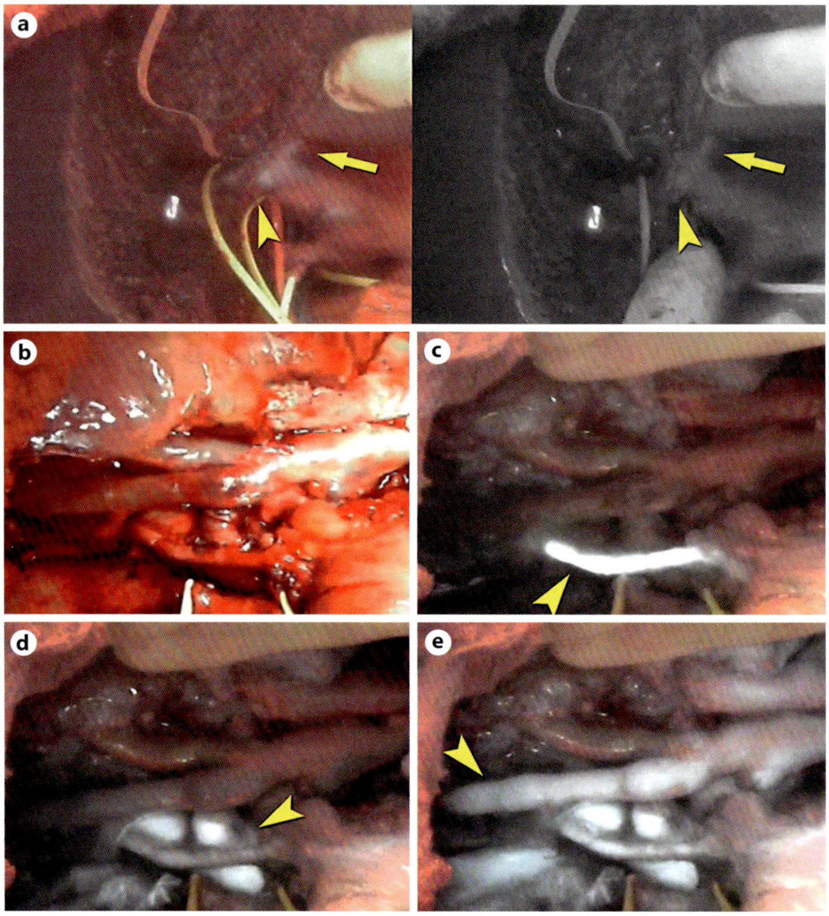

Fig. 1. Fluorescence cholangiography and angiography in LDLT. **a** The fluorescence image (right) is overlaid on the color image (left). The fluorescence image of the confluence of the left (arrowhead) and right (arrow) hepatic ducts is clearly delineated with the color images of the surrounding structures. **b** Intraoperative gross appearance of the right liver graft transplanted in a LDLT recipient after the reconstruction of the hepatic vessels. **c** Fluorescence imaging following intravenous injection of ICG delineates continuous blood flow through the anastomosis between the right hepatic arteries (arrowhead). **d** Following the arteriography, the portal venous flow (arrowhead) is visualized. **e** Finally, fluorescence imaging identifies hepatic venous flow through the cryopreserved vein graft (arrowhead), which is used for the reconstruction of the middle hepatic vein tributaries.

fluorescence imaging systems that reveal biological structures with fluorescence of ICG only on monochromatic images. In contrast, fluorescence cholangiography is limited in its ability to delineate deeply located hepatic ducts since the tissue penetration ability of ICG fluorescence is limited to 5–10 mm [4]. Concomitant use of conventional radiographic cholangiography is needed to confirm the anatomy of the intrahepatic bile ducts during donor surgery.

Fluorescence Angiography for Recipient Surgery

Background

Originally, fluorescence angiography using ICG was used to assess coronary artery bypass graft patency during cardiac surgery [11, 12]. This technique was first applied to LDLT procedures by Kubota et al. [13], with the aim of evaluating blood flow through anastomoses of both the hepatic arteries and portal veins. The authors' group also used fluorescence angiography in recipient surgery using the subsequent imaging system, which enabled simultaneous visualization of ICG fluorescence on the color images [3].

Administration of Indocyanine Green

Intraoperative fluorescence angiography is performed by intravenous injection of 1 ml ICG (2.5 mg).

Visualization of Hepatic Blood Flow after Venous Reconstruction

After procurement of the liver graft and reconstruction of the hepatic vessels, fluorescent imaging enables visualization of continuous arterial blood flow, portal venous flow and hepatic venous flow following intravenous injection of ICG. Figure 1b–e shows fluorescence images of hepatic blood flow after vessel reconstructions in LDLT using a right liver graft. Fluorescence imaging using the HyperEye Medical System delineates continuous blood flow through the anastomotic site between the right hepatic arteries and portal veins, and finally the hepatic venous flow in cryopreserved vein grafts, which was used for the reconstruction of the stumps of the middle hepatic vein tributaries.

Evaluation of the Portal Uptake Function

Background

Venous occlusion in the remnant liver after resection or in the graft in LDLT can make the portal veins function as drainage vessels [14], resulting in necrosis [15] or insufficient regeneration [16] of such veno-occlusive regions, which can cause severe difficulty in postoperative management [17, 18]. In order to prevent postoperative hepatic dysfunction in veno-occlusive regions, stumps of the major hepatic vein tributaries are sometimes reconstructed during liver resection [19] and LDLT [20, 21], especially when the remnant liver volume is estimated to be insufficient based on the calculation using preoperative computed tomography (CT). However, it has been unclear to what extent the liver function in such veno-occlusive hepatic regions might decrease.

Hashimoto et al. [22] first reported a technique for the evaluation of sinusoidal perfusion in veno-occlusive regions in the remnant liver after graft procurement, using intraoperative ICG injection and near-infrared spectroscopy. However, their technique is somewhat complex for intraoperative evaluation in clinical settings and

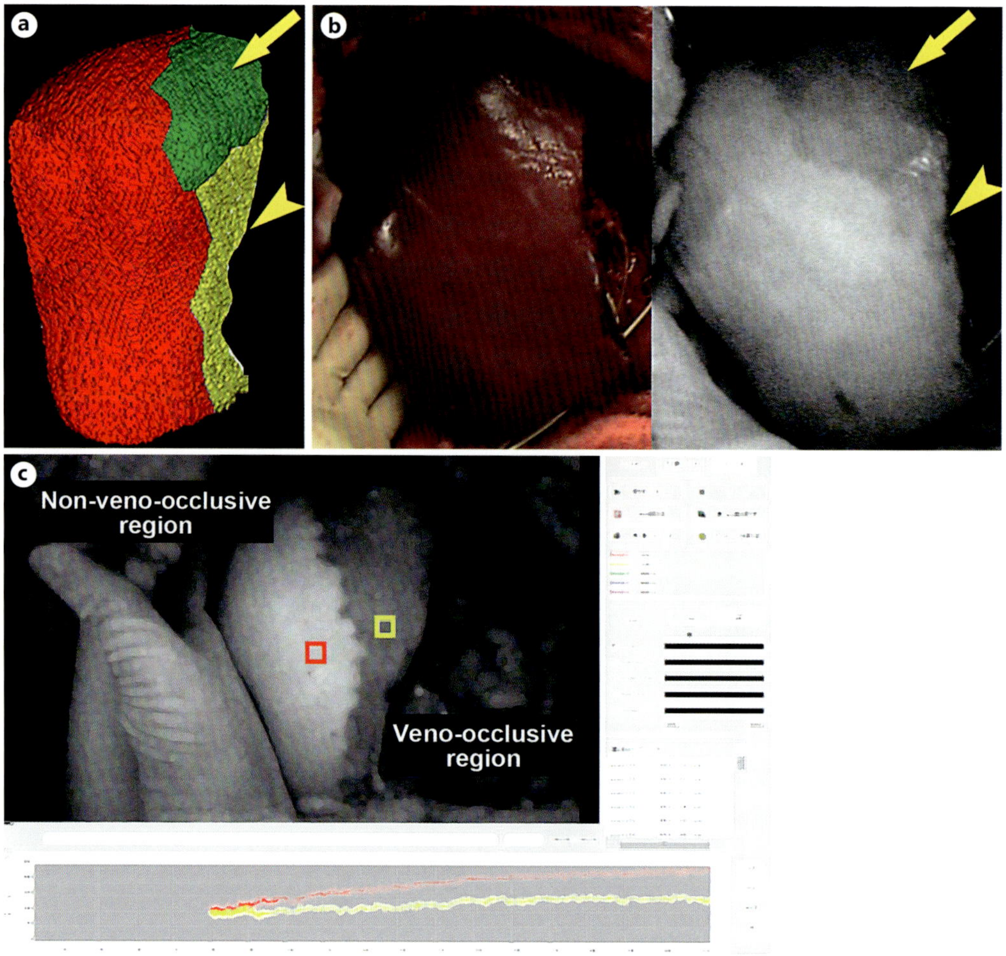

Fig. 2. Evaluation of the portal uptake function in veno-occlusive hepatic regions by intraoperative ICG fluorescence imaging. **a** Preoperative 3D reconstruction of CT images reveals hepatic regions drained by the right hepatic vein (red) and middle hepatic vein tributaries draining segment VIII (green) and segment V (yellow) in the right liver graft. **b** Intraoperative fluorescence imaging following intravenous injection of ICG reveals the difference in the distributions of ICG between veno-occlusive regions. The left picture shows the gross appearance of the right liver graft after reconstruction of the hepatic artery, portal vein and hepatic veins (right hepatic vein, middle hepatic vein and middle hepatic vein tributaries draining segments VIII and V). **c** By using a luminance-analyzing software, intersegmental changes in the fluorescence intensity, which reflect the distribution of ICG after intravenous injection, can be evaluated quantitatively.

has limitations in demonstrating the intersegmental difference in the portal uptake function at the same time. Recently, the authors' group improved their technique for evaluation of the liver function in veno-occlusive regions by evaluating the fluorescence intensities of hepatic regions using a fluorescence imaging system in real time during surgery, as described below [23].

Administration of ICG
Intraoperatively, ICG (2.5 μg per 1 ml of remnant liver volume calculated based on the preoperative CT) is administered intravenously following division of the major hepatic vein tributaries or the reconstruction of hepatic vessels [23].

Intraoperative Evaluation of the Portal Uptake Function in Veno-Occlusive Regions
Following the intravenous injection of ICG, fluorescence images of the liver surface are obtained using a commercially available fluorescence imaging system (PDE; Hamamatsu Photonics, Hamamatsu, Japan) for approximately 5 min. Then, the extent of decrease in the portal uptake function due to venous occlusion can be visualized as a difference in the fluorescence intensities among hepatic segments (fig. 2a). In order to quantitate the segmental portal uptake function, the fluorescence intensity values can be calculated using a luminance-analyzing software (U11437, Hamamatsu Photonics). In our previous series consisting of patients undergoing liver resection and LDLT donors and recipients, the portal uptake function in veno-occlusive regions is approximately 30–40% of that in the veno-occlusive regions [23]. Such information on the portal uptake function in veno-occlusive liver obtained by ICG fluorescence imaging would be helpful for surgeons to decide the indication of liver resection or LDLT before surgery and to determine the need for venous reconstruction intraoperatively.

Conclusions

ICG fluorescence imaging can be utilized during liver transplantation not only to visualize the bile duct anatomy and blood flow after venous reconstructions, but also to evaluate the portal uptake function in veno-occlusive hepatic regions, enhancing the accuracy and safety of surgery.

References

1 Mitsuhashi N, Kimura F, Shimizu H, et al: Usefulness of intraoperative fluorescence imaging to evaluate local anatomy in hepatobiliary surgery. J Hepatobiliary Pancreat Surg 2008;15:508–514.
2 Ishizawa T, Bandai Y, Ijichi M, et al: Fluorescent cholangiography illuminating the biliary tree during laparoscopic cholecystectomy. Br J Surg 2010;97: 1369–1377.
3 Kawaguchi Y, Ishizawa T, Masuda K, et al: Hepatobiliary surgery guided by a novel fluorescent imaging technique for visualizing hepatic arteries, bile ducts, and liver cancers on color images. J Am Coll Surg 2011;212:e33–e39.
4 Ishizawa T, Fukushima N, Shibahara J, et al: Realtime identification of liver cancers by using indocyanine green fluorescent imaging. Cancer 2009;115: 2491–2504.
5 Gotoh K, Yamada T, Ishikawa O, et al: A novel image-guided surgery of hepatocellular carcinoma by indocyanine green fluorescence imaging navigation. J Surg Oncol 2009;100:75–79.
6 Aoki T, Murakami M, Yasuda D, et al: Intraoperative fluorescent imaging using indocyanine green for liver mapping and cholangiography. J Hepatobiliary Pancreat Sci 2010;17:590–594.

7 Harada N, Ishizawa T, Muraoka A, et al: Fluorescence navigation hepatectomy by visualization of localized cholestasis from bile duct tumor infiltration. J Am Coll Surg 2010;210:e2–e6.
8 Cattral MS, Greig PD, Muradali D, et al: Reconstruction of middle hepatic vein of a living-donor right lobe liver graft with recipient left portal vein. Transplantation 2001;71:1864–1866.
9 Sano K, Makuuchi M, Miki K, et al: Evaluation of hepatic venous congestion: proposed indication criteria for hepatic vein reconstruction. Ann Surg 2002; 236:241–247.
10 Ishizawa T, Tamura S, Masuda K, et al: Intraoperative fluorescent cholangiography using indocyanine green: a biliary road map for safe surgery. J Am Coll Surg 2009;208:e1–e4.
11 Rubens FD, Ruel M, Fremes SE: A new and simplified method for coronary and graft imaging during CABG. Heart Surg Forum 2002;5:141–144.
12 Taggart DP, Choudhary B, Anastasiadis K, et al: Preliminary experience with a novel intraoperative fluorescence imaging technique to evaluate the patency of bypass grafts in total arterial revascularization. Ann Thorac Surg 2003;75:870–873.
13 Kubota K, Kita J, Shimoda M, et al: Intraoperative assessment of reconstructed vessels in living-donor liver transplantation, using a novel fluorescence imaging technique. J Hepatobiliary Pancreat Surg 2006; 13:100–104.
14 Murata S, Itai Y, Asato M, Kobayashi H, et al: Effect of temporary occlusion of the hepatic vein on dual blood in the liver: evaluation with spiral CT. Radiology 1995;197:351–356.
15 Lee S, Park K, Hwang S, et al: Congestion of right liver graft in living donor liver transplantation. Transplantation 2001;71:812–814.
16 Akamatsu N, Sugawara Y, Kaneko J, et al: Effects of middle hepatic vein reconstruction on right liver graft regeneration. Transplantation 2003;76:832–837.
17 Buell JF, Funaki B, Cronin DC, et al: Long-term venous complications after full-size and segmental pediatric liver transplantation. Ann Surg 2002;236: 658–666.
18 Akamatsu N, Sugawara Y, Kaneko J, et al: Surgical repair for late-onset hepatic venous outflow block after living-donor liver transplantation. Transplantation 2004;77:1768–1770.
19 Kakazu T, Makuuchi M, Kawasaki S, et al: Reconstruction of the middle hepatic vein tributary during right anterior segmentectomy. Surgery 1995;117: 238–240.
20 Cattral MS, Greig PD, Muradali D, Grant D: Reconstruction of middle hepatic vein of a living-donor right lobe liver graft with recipient left portal vein. Transplantation 2001;71:1864–1866.
21 Sano K, Makuuchi M, Miki K, et al: Evaluation of hepatic venous congestion: proposed indication criteria for hepatic vein reconstruction. Ann Surg 2002; 236:241–247.
22 Hashimoto T, Miki K, Imamura H, et al: Sinusoidal perfusion in the veno-occlusive region of living liver donors evaluated by indocyanine green and near-infrared spectroscopy. Liver Transpl 2008;14:872–880.
23 Kawaguchi Y, Ishizawa T, Miyata Y, et al: Portal uptake function in veno-occlusive regions evaluated by real-time fluorescent imaging using indocyanine green. J Hepatol 2013;58:247–253.

Norihiro Kokudo, MD, PhD
Hepato-Biliary-Pancreatic Surgery Division, Department of Surgery
Graduate School of Medicine, The University of Tokyo
7-3-1 Hongo, Bunkyo-ku, Tokyo 113-8655 (Japan)
E-Mail KOKUDO-2SU@h.u-tokyo.ac.jp

Kokudo N, Ishizawa T (eds): Fluorescent Imaging: Treatment of Hepatobiliary and Pancreatic Diseases.
Front Gastrointest Res. Basel, Karger, 2013, vol 31, pp 49–57 (DOI: 10.1159/000348606)

Staining of Liver Segments

Takeshi Aoki[a] · Mashiko Murakami[a] · Mitsuo Kusano[b]

[a]Department of Surgery, School of Medicine, Showa University, Tokyo, and
[b]Kushiro Rosai Hospital, Hokkaido, Japan

Abstract

Anatomic hepatic segmentectomy is considered the gold standard approach for liver resection in patients with hepatocellular carcinoma, with the goal of reducing cancer recurrence after liver resection. This approach may also be useful for other indications, such as for segmental resection of colorectal metastases and other hepatic tumors. Thus, identification of liver segments is crucial for segment-oriented surgical resection. The classic hepatic segment identification technique involves puncture of a segmental portal branch under the guidance of intraoperative ultrasonography. Recently, a fluorescence imaging technique utilizing indocyanine green (ICG) as a fluorescence source has been developed and applied to hepatobiliary surgery for intraoperative visualization of the hepatic segment, bile duct and liver cancers. In this chapter, we describe a novel method for the clear demarcation of the resection area by means of ICG fluorescence with a light-emitting diode camera system to systematically accomplish anatomic segmental and subsegmental resections.

Anatomical resection can improve survival and limit complications from hepatectomy in patients with hepatocellular carcinoma (HCC). Because of the high likelihood of cancer cells from HCC spreading through the portal venous system and causing intrahepatic metastases [1–3], anatomic resection may be more effective for eradication of intrahepatic metastases of HCC when compared with nonanatomical resection. Thus, intraoperative identification of liver segments remains essential for segment-oriented surgical resection.

Mapping with vital blue dyes under intraoperative ultrasound (IOUS) is currently the gold standard for identifying segments and subsegments in the liver [1]. However, this method can sometimes yield indistinct results, and it is much more difficult to reproduce these procedures laparoscopically and confirm the demarcation of the hepatic segment visually. Hence, development of new or additional intraoperative imaging strategies would be of benefit.

Illumination with near-infrared light has recently been employed to detect sentinel lymph nodes in the context of breast [4, 5], gastric [6, 7], lung [8, 9] and esophageal cancers [10], and to intraoperatively assess graft patency [11–16]. Fluorescent navigation surgery is increasingly being used to identify sentinel lymph nodes in cancers of the breast and digestive organs, and also to detect cerebral vessels and coronary arteries. We previously demonstrated that indocyanine green (ICG) fluorescence imaging is extremely useful to achieve clear demarcation of liver segments [17]. Moreover, fluorescence intraoperative cholangiography using ICG is a safe and valuable method of characterizing the biliary tract anatomy [18–20]. These techniques are based on the finding that ICG binds to plasma proteins and that protein-bound ICG emits light with a peak wavelength of around 830 nm when excited with near-infrared light.

In this chapter, we describe an intraoperative method for the identification of liver segments using a highly sensitive ICG fluorescence imaging system.

Fluorescence Imaging System

Fluorescence imaging is performed by injection of ICG (Diagnogreen; Daiichi Sankyo Co., Tokyo, Japan), and our institution utilizes the so-called Photodynamic Eye (PDE) fluorescence imaging system from Hamamatsu Photonics (Hamamatsu, Japan) [18, 19]. The light source is a light-emitting diode, emitting light at a wavelength of 760 nm, and the detector is a charge-coupled device camera that subsequently filters out light with wavelengths <820 nm. A total of 36 light-emitting diodes are aligned on a board in an area, with the charge-coupled device camera set in the center. Fluorescence signals are sent to a digital video processor for display on a monitor. Using this system, ICG bound to human plasma is detectable as a fluorescence signal by an infrared observation camera system (fig. 1).

Another fluorescence imaging system (HyperEye Medical System; Mizuho Ikakogyo Co. Ltd., Tokyo, Japan) is also useful for identifying fluorescence signals during liver surgery [19, 20]. The camera unit of this system is equipped with optical filters and a highly sensitive charge-coupled device camera with a 10× optical zoom, which enables visualization of both visible and near-infrared rays using a selector switch [21].

Identification of Liver Segments and Subsegments by Indocyanine Green Fluorescence

We previously reported that liver segments can be identified by injection of 1 ml of ICG (5 mg/ml; Diagnogreen) via a 23-gauge needle into the portal vein branch with a Pringle maneuver under ultrasonography. However, a recent study demonstrated that a much more diluted concentration of ICG (i.e. 0.025 mg in 10 ml of normal saline) was sufficient to produce a clear demarcation line in the liver [21]. An inter-

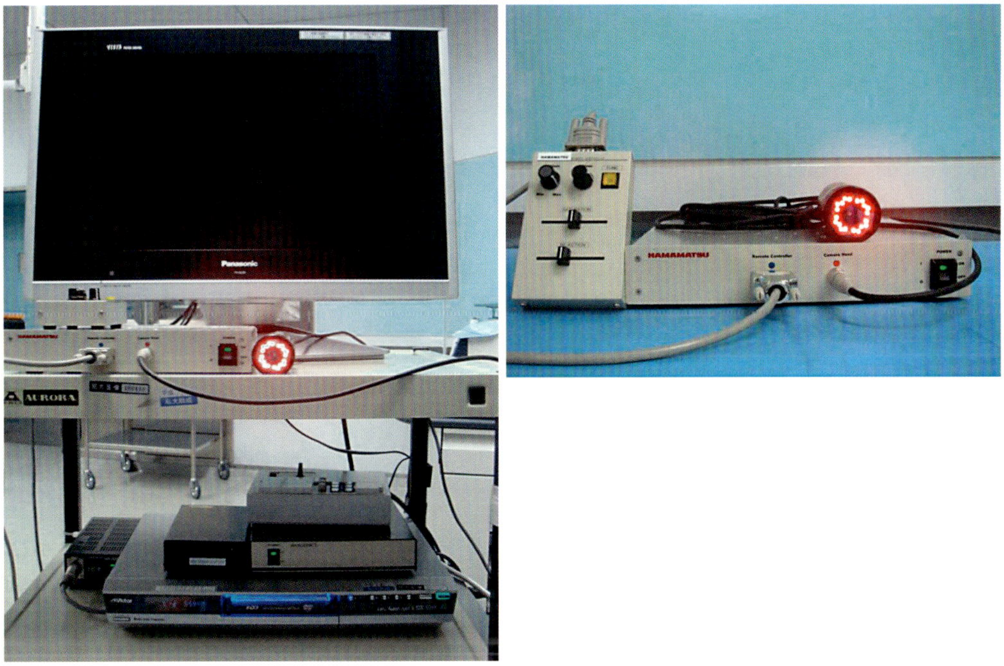

Fig. 1. Fluorescence imaging system (PDE; Hamamatsu Photonics) including a charge-coupled device camera.

mittent Pringle maneuver required periods of inflow clamping (15 min) for the injection of ICG to avoid fluorescence of whole liver.

The PDE infrared observation camera system was linked to the fluorescence excitation of ICG by light-emitting diodes immediately after the operating room was darkened. The fluorescence signals were transmitted to a digital video processor and displayed on a TV monitor in real time. At this point, the extent of liver segments and subsegments can be determined according to the results of dye injection through the portal vein.

Anatomical Hepatic Resection Guided by the Indocyanine Green Fluorescence Imaging System

The surgical procedures used in our institution for hepatic resections guided by the ICG fluorescence system are summarized in table 1. Stained subsegments and segments of the liver were identifiable in 33 (94.3%) of 35 patients using the PDE. The development of collaterals in cirrhotic patients with high portal pressure results in portal systemic shunting, which may interfere with staining by ICG. In our series, the procedure was unsuccessful due to blockage of portal flow secondary to portal hypertension in one patient and due to technical failure with the injection in another patient

Table 1. Detection rate of demarcation of the liver segment using ICG fluorescence

Liver type		Complications
cirrhotic	noncirrhotic	
13/15 (86.6%)	60/66 (90.9%)	0/81

with liver cirrhosis. However, there was no significant difference between noncirrhotic livers and cirrhotic livers in terms of demarcation of the hepatic segments (table 1). There were no problems with the PDE during operation. No postoperative complications or adverse effects related to the injection of ICG were observed.

Mapping of Liver Segments

Liver segments were not consistently visualized by all attending surgeons in response to the use of ICG alone, whereas segments and subsegments of the liver were immediately and distinctly identified with the PDE camera system 1 min after ICG injection. The demarcation line of a liver segment or subsegment was distinguished with fluorescence and the PDE, even 10 min after injection. Figure 2 shows the demarcation of segment VII, which is clearly identified under PDE observation. Thus, demarcation of liver subsegments was readily achieved using electrocautery (fig. 2).

Counterstaining Method for Mapping of Liver Segments

Recently, Ishizawa et al. [22] reported that negative staining of hepatic segments using fluorescence imaging techniques during laparoscopic hepatectomy enabled identification of hepatic segments prior to and during parenchymal transection. This staining method was simple and useful to visually confirm demarcation of the hepatic segment on the monitor during laparoscopic liver surgery and was achieved by intravenously administering ICG dye after clamping the segmental portal pedicle.

Figure 3a shows negative staining of the segment IV inferior for resection in a patient with HCC. The root of the portal pedicle for segment IV inferior was temporarily clamped and 1 ml of ICG dye (5 mg/dl) was intravenously injected via a central vein. All hepatic segments, except for segment IV inferior, had clear fluorescence 1 min after injection, and the area border was easily marked for resection. Figure 3b shows a case in which an 18-gauge microwave coagulating therapy needle was inserted into the portal branch near the tumor in segment VI. This was visualized under IOUS and was done to ablate the feeding portal and arterial branches. Subsequently,

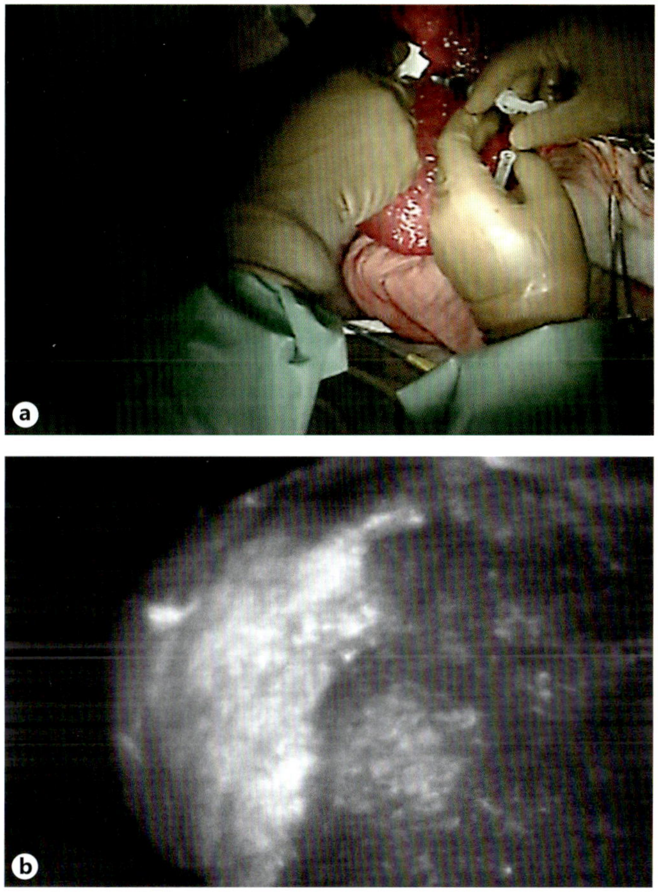

Fig. 2. a Green staining of the liver surface after injection of ICG via the portal vein is not visualized clearly. **b** After injection of fluorescent ICG, Segment VII is clearly demonstrated using the fluorescence imaging system.

1 ml of ICG was intravenously injected via a central vein. Negative fluorescent staining was observed on the liver surface, and a line for surgical removal of the area of nonfluorescence was determined. This counterstaining method via intravenous administration of ICG after the occluding of the segmental branches of vessels was easy to perform and effective for identifying the demarcation of liver segment.

Discussion

Because of the pattern of intrahepatic spread of HCC, anatomic segmental liver resection is considered to be the gold standard to reduce the recurrence of the tumor. However, anatomic subsegmental resection is a demanding procedure and requires adequate skill in ultrasound exploration. Makuuchi et al. [1] described a puncture technique under IOUS guidance followed by injection of ICG into the vessel while the hepatic artery at the hepatic hilum was clamped; this enabled the portal branch feed-

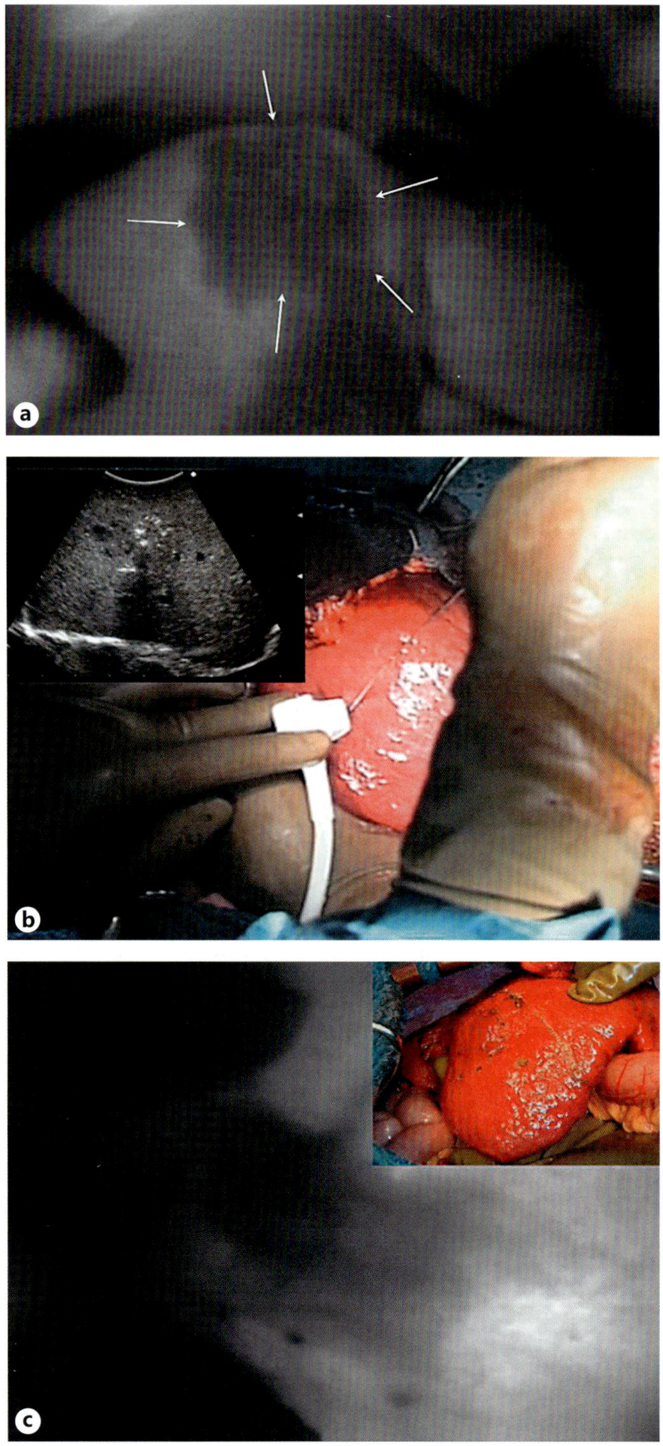

Fig. 3. a After clamping the root of the portal pedicle for segment IV inferior, ICG dye was intravenously injected via a central vein. All hepatic segments, except for segment IV inferior, are clearly fluorescent. This enables determination of the surgical line for removal of the area of non fluorescence. **b** After ablating the feeding portal and arterial branches, 1 ml of ICG was intravenously injected via a central vein. **c** Negative fluorescent staining of segment VI inferior was observed on the liver surface.

ing the tumor to be resected after puncture. The stained area was evident on the liver surface, the area was marked with electrocautery, and the hepatic artery was then unclamped. Although the liver segment can be easily detected when using this technique, hepatic artery clamping is recommended. In comparison, hepatic artery clamping is not required in the ICG technique because the ICG dye is taken up by hepatocytes of the segment to be stained immediately after injection into the portal branch. Another simple method is the glissonian pedicle approach, which can separate the liver into three sections by simply clamping the secondary glissonian pedicle extrahepatically without liver dissection at the hepatic hilus [23, 24]. This technique can be difficult in patients with insufficient liver function, who require smaller anatomical resection, such as cone unit resection, because a high skill level is necessary to detect the tertiary branches. The ICG fluorescence technique, however, is a simple and quick method that can identify the clear demarcation of the liver segment or subsegment in patients with insufficient liver function, such as liver cirrhosis. Other techniques to enable precise anatomical liver segmental resection have been proposed, such as the use of a balloon catheter inserted transhepatically to occlude the feeding portal branch [25]. For segment VIII resection, Mazziotti et al. [26] proposed division of the liver along the main portal fissure and an intraparenchymal approach to the segment VIII glissonian pedicle. However, these techniques are an invasive approach to identify the demarcation of the liver segment. Recently, Torzilli et al. [27] described ultrasound-guided finger compression subsegmentectomy for detection of liver segments. Although this technique is a simple and safe way to identify the demarcation of liver in open liver surgery, it may be difficult to handle IOUS during laparoscopic liver surgery for the purposes of achieving clear demarcation of the liver segments. In comparison to the IOUS-guided technique, the ICG fluorescence imaging technique has two options to image the liver segment: injecting ICG dye into the segmental portal branch under guidance of IOUS, or by intravenously administering ICG dye after clamping the segmental portal pedicle. Thus, the individual staining method for identification of liver segment can be selected according to the type of the operation. For example, the ICG fluorescence imaging technique is suitable for accurate anatomical laparoscopic hepatic resection with the assistance of hepatic segment imaging following intravenous administration of ICG after clamping the segmental portal pedicle [22].

ICG has excitation (800 nm) and fluorescence (840 nm) wavelengths in the near-infrared range when it binds to plasma proteins, such as high-density lipoprotein and low-density lipoprotein. Near-infrared light penetrates deeply into living tissues. Thus, ICG fluorescence imaging has an advantage of being compatible with the biochemical characteristics of living tissues. We previously reported that the fluorescence imaging technique was safe and reproducible, and that it provided insights for either subsegmentectomy or segmentectomy in patients with a malignant hepatic neoplasm [17, 18]. Moreover, this method enables the visualization of hepatic segments during liver surgery following intravenous administration of ICG after clamping the segmental portal pedicle [22]. Ishizawa et al. [22] demonstrated that ICG fluorescence enabled visualization of hepatic segments during laparoscopic surgery by intravenously administering ICG after clamping the portal pedicle (negative staining). The negative-staining technique was easy and most appropriate for the resection of left segments or inferior segments in which the roots of these segmental portal branches were easily approached. During laparoscopic liver resection, it is more difficult to handle IOUS to confirm demarcation of the hepatic segment visually on the monitor when compared with open liver surgery. To overcome this problem, intravenous administration of ICG after clamping the portal pedicle (negative staining) has the advantages of being simple and facilitating accurate laparoscopic anatomical segmentectomy. In regard to anatomical liver resection using ICG fluorescence, Uchiyama et al. [28] advocated the combined use of a ICG fluorescence navigation system and contrast-enhanced intraoperative ultrasonography image using Sonazoid™, a novel modality for the detection of liver sections and segments during anatomical hepatic resection. These observations suggest that the ICG fluorescence technique effectively enables accurate anatomical hepatic resection with the assistance of hepatic segment imaging.

In conclusion, staining of the liver using ICG and infrared light enables safe and effective segmental hepatectomy for patients with liver neoplasm.

References

1 Makuuchi M, Hasegawa H, Yamazaki S, et al: Ultrasonically guided subsegmentectomy. Surg Gynecol Obset 1986;126:346–350.

2 Makino I, Chijiiwa K, Kondo K, et al: Prognostic benefit of selective portal vein occulusion during hepatic resection for hepatocellualr carcinoma. Surgery 2005;137:626–631.

3 Hasegawa K, Kokudo N, Imamura H, et al: Prognostic impact of anatomic resection for hepatocellular carcinoma. Ann Surg 2005;242:252–259.

4 Kitai T, ItamotoT, Miwa M, et al: Fluorescence navigation with indocyanine green for detecting sentinel lymph nodes in breast cancer. Breast Cancer 2005;12:211–215.

5 Motomura K, Inaji H, Komoike Y, et al: Sentinel node biopsy guided by indocyanine green dye in breast cancer patients. Jpn J Clin Oncol 1999;29:604–607.

6 Nimura H, Narimiya N, Mitsumori N, et al: Infrared ray electronic endoscopy combined with indocyanine green injection for detection of sentinel nodes of patients with gastric cancer. Br J Surg 2004;91:575–579.

7 Ishikawa K, Yasuda K, Shiromizu A, et al: Laparoscopic sentinel node navigation achieved by infrared ray electronic endoscopy system in patients with gastric cancer. Surg Endosc 2007;21:1131–1134.

8 Ito N, Fukuta M, Tokushima T, et al: Sentinel node navigation surgery using indocyanine green in patients with lung cancer. Surg Today 2004;34:581–585.

9 Soltesz EG, Kim S, Laurence RG, et al: Intraoperative sentinel lymph node mapping of the lung using near-infrared fluorescent quantum dots. Ann Thorac Surg 2005;79:269–277.

10 Parungo CP, Ohnishi S, Kim SW, et al: Intraoperative identification of esophageal sentinel lymph nodes with near infrared fluorescence imaging. J Thorac Cardiovasc Surg 2005;129:844–850.

11 Taggart DP, Choudhary B, Anastasiadis K, et al: Preliminary experience with a novel intraoperative fluorescence imaging technique to evaluate the patency of bypass grafts in total arterial revascularization. Ann Thorac Surg 2003;75:870–873.

12 Detter C, Russ D, Iffand A, et al: Near-infrared fluorescence coronary angiography: a new noninvasive technology for intraoperative graft patency control. Heart Surg Forum 2002;5:364–369.

13 Rubens FD, Ruel M, Fremes SE, et al: A new and simplified method for coronary and graft imaging during CABG. Heart Surg Forum 2002;5:141–144.

14 Sekijima M, Tojimbara T, Sato S, et al: An intraoperative fluorescent imaging system in organ transplantation. Transplant Proc 2004;36:2188–2190.

15 Raabe A, Beck J, Gerlach R, et al: Near-infrared indocyanine green video angiography: a new method for intraoperative assessment of vascular flow. Neurosurgery 2003;52:132–139.
16 Kuroiwa T, Kajimoto Y, Ohta T: Development and clinical application of near-infrared surgical microscope: preliminary report. Minim Invasive Neurosurg 2001;44:240–242.
17 Aoki T, Yasuda D, Shimizu Y, et al: Image-guided liver mapping using fluorescence navigation system with indocyanine green for anatomical hepatic resection. World J Surg 2008;32:1763–1767.
18 Aoki T, Murakami M, Yasuda D, et al: Intraoperative fluorescent imaging using indocyanine green for liver mapping and chorangiography. J Hepatobiliary Pancret Sci 2010;17:590–594.
19 Ishizawa T, Tamura S, Masuda K, Aoki T, Hasegawa K, Imamura H, Beck Y, Kokudo N: Intraopearative fluorescent cholangiography using indocyanine green: a biliary road map for safe surgery. J Am Coll Surg 2008;208:e1–e4.
20 Ishizawa T, Bandai Y, Kokudo N: Fluorescent cholangiography using indocyanine green for laparoscopic cholecystectomy: an initial experience. Arch Surg 2009;144:381–382.
21 Kawaguchi Y, Ishizawa T, Masuda K, et al: Hepatobiliary surgery guided by a novel fluorescent imaging technique for visualizing hepatic arteries, bile duct, and liver cancers on color images. J Am Coll Surg 2011;212:e33–e39.
22 Ishizawa T, Zuker NB, Kokudo N, Gayet B: Positive and negative staining of hepatic segments by use of fluorescent imaging techniques during laparoscopic hepatectomy. Arch Surg 2012;147:393–394.
23 Takasaki K: Glissonean pedicle transection method for hepatic resection: a new concept of liver segmentation. J Hepatobiliary Pancreat Surg 1998;5:286–291.
24 Yamamoto M, Katagiri S, Arizumi S, Kotera Y, Takahashi Y: Glissonean pedicle transection method for liver surgery. J Hepatobiliary Panceat Sci 2012;19:3–8.
25 Shimamura Y, Gunven P, Takenaka Y, et al: Selective portal branch occlusion by balloon catheter during liver resection. Surgery 1986;100:938–941.
26 Mazziotti A, Maeda A, Ercolani G, et al: Isolated resection of segment 8 for liver tumors: a new approach for anatomical segmentectomy. Arch Surg 2000;135:1224–1229.
27 Torzilli G, Procopio F, Cimino M, et al: Anatomical segmental and subsegmental resection of the liver for hepatocellular carcinoma: a new approach by means of ultrasound-guided vessel compression. Ann Surg 2010;251:229–235.
28 Uchiyama K, Ueno M, Ozawa S, et al: Combined intraoperative use of contrast-enhanced ultrasonography imaging using a sonazoid and fluorescence navigation system with indocyanine green during anatomical hepatectomy. Langenbecks Arch Surg 2011:396:1101–1107.

Takeshi Aoki
Department of Surgery, School of Medicine
Showa University, 1-5-8 Hatanodai, Shinagawaku
Tokyo 142-8666 (Japan)
E-Mail takejp@wb4.so-net.ne.jp

Kokudo N, Ishizawa T (eds): Fluorescent Imaging: Treatment of Hepatobiliary and Pancreatic Diseases.
Front Gastrointest Res. Basel, Karger, 2013, vol 31, pp 58–65 (DOI: 10.1159/000348608)

Visualization of Cholecystic Venous Flow for Hepatic Resection in Gallbladder Carcinoma

Kyohei Kai

Department of Surgery, Japanese Red Cross Society Himeji Hospital, Himeji, Japan

Abstract

It is well-known that some hepatic resection is required in T2 gallbladder carcinoma to ensure that microscopic metastases around the gallbladder bed are excised, but the appropriate extent of hepatic resection has not been established. Based on the results of clinical and pathological studies, hepatic wedge resection is currently performed 1–2 cm distant from the gallbladder bed; however, it is unclear whether this area is sufficient in each individual patient. We have developed the following technique using fluorescence angiography to determine the necessary extent of resection: indocyanine green is injected into the cholecystic artery, and cholecystic venous flow is then observed using a near-infrared camera system. This highly sensitive technique enables us to evaluate blood flow in real time. We classified fluorescence patterns into two types according to the site and timing of fluorescence. In type 1, cholecystic veins flow directly into the liver parenchyma adjacent to the gallbladder. In type 2, cholecystic veins flow into intraportal branches. We propose that the type 1 pathway is the main route of hepatic metastasis in early advanced gallbladder carcinoma. Sufficient hepatic resection around the gallbladder bed, whether anatomical or nonanatomical, is needed to prevent recurrence in the remnant liver. Using our newly developed fluorescence angiography technique, we now perform hepatic resection according to the cholecystic venous perfusion area.

Hepatic and lymph node metastases increase in frequency once gallbladder carcinoma reaches the subserosa. It is well known that the most likely site of hepatic metastasis in patients with advanced gallbladder carcinoma is within the S4a or S5 segment [1–3], as defined by Couinaud's segmental nomenclature. The purpose of hepatic resection in gallbladder carcinoma is to macroscopically and microscopically remove the liver parenchyma containing metastatic lesions. Advanced gallbladder carcinoma involving the liver parenchyma may require extensive hepatic resection, depending on the extent of liver involvement. Partial hepatic resection with lymph node dissection is regarded as the standard procedure in T2 gallbladder carcinoma [4–7]; however, the appropriate extent of resection has not yet been established. The limitation of partial hepatic resection is because of the lack of definite anatomical landmarks; the range of hepatic resection therefore differs subtly from center to center. The primary purpose of this chapter is to explain how to determine the extent of hepatic resection necessary in T2 gallbladder carcinoma. Our newly developed fluorescence angiography technique makes it possible to determine the appropriate site and extent of hepatectomy according to the cholecystic venous perfusion area.

Route of Hepatic Metastasis in Gallbladder Carcinoma

Recent pathological studies have demonstrated that the main metastatic route of gallbladder carcinoma is lymphatic spread within the portal tract [1, 2]. Shirai et al. [1] examined the gross and histological patterns of hepatic metastasis in 20 resected specimens and classified the mode of hepatic spread into the following three patterns: (1) direct invasion through the gallbladder bed, (2) microscopic angiolymphatic invasion of portal tracts, and (3) distant hepatic metastatic nodules. They suggested that microscopic angiolymphatic lesions are found within 20 mm of the direct-invasion tumor border; furthermore, they emphasized that lymphatic spread within the portal tract is the driving force behind hepatic spread. In an experimental pig model, Terazawa et al. [8] examined the lymphatic flow using the carbon particle suspension CH40 and the contrast agent Lipiodol. When the lymphatic drainage route is occluded at Calot's triangle, thereby interrupting the normal lymphatic flow, the agents spread into the liver parenchyma adjacent to the gallbladder.

These findings seem to provide an explanation for the high incidence of micrometastases surrounding the gallbladder bed, although these theories of lymphatic spread are inconsistent. Shirai et al. [1] suggested that distant hepatic nodules (pattern 3) are likely to be of hematogenous origin, with hematogenous spread playing a minor role in hepatic metastasis dissemination. They suggest that the pattern of some metastatic lesions in the liver corresponds to the lymphatic pathway, with the pattern of other lesions corresponding to the hematogenous pathway. Their experimental results, however, do not necessarily show that lymphatic spread is the main route for the dissemination of hepatic metastases. Lymphatic fluid does not flow from the gallbladder to the liver parenchyma under normal conditions, meaning that lymphatic flow may not be responsible for hepatic metastasis in early-stage gallbladder carcinoma.

Studies using computed tomography angiography (CTA) have suggested that the cholecystic venous flow is closely related to the pattern of hepatic metastasis [9], thereby representing an important metastatic route [10]. Studies using this modality have demonstrated that the cholecystic venous flow drains directly into the sinusoids of the liver. Ohtani et al. [11] traced fluid pathways from the hepatic sinusoids to the interstitial space of the portal tracts, and finally to the lymphatic vessels. Cancerous cells in the sinusoids, delivered there by the cholecystic veins, may therefore reach lymphatic vessels through this pathway. Shirai et al. [1] and Ohtsuka et al. [2] described lymphatic spread along the portal tract, but their pathological findings show that cancer cells are present in the interstitial space of the portal tract and the portal lymphatic vessels. The hematogenous spread theory may provide a consistent explanation of how cancer cells spread into the liver parenchyma in early-stage gallbladder carcinoma, finally reaching lymphatic vessels along the portal tract.

Fluorescence Angiography

We evaluated cholecystic venous flow using a newly developed, minimally invasive fluorescence angiography technique, requiring superselective catheterization of the cholecystic artery [12]. In this technique, we injected indocyanine green (ICG) (Diagnogreen; Daiichi Pharmaceutical Co., Tokyo, Japan) directly into the cholecystic artery and observed the cholecystic venous flow using a near-infrared camera system. This technique is highly sensitive, enabling us to observe the blood flow in real time.

Laparotomy was performed under general anesthesia. To avoid arterial spasm, 1 ml of 1% lidocaine was injected around the cholecystic artery at Calot's triangle. Particular attention was directed toward cholecystic vein injury because normal cholecystic venous perfusion may be affected by injured vessels. After superselective cannulation of the cholecystic artery, a small volume (0.5 ml) of diluted ICG was slowly injected. A larger volume of ICG should be avoided because it may result in excitation of the entire liver surface. A light-emitting diode was then used to excite fluorescence in ICG combined with plasma proteins; the peak fluorescence value was 860 nm. A Photodynamic Eye (PDE; Hamamatsu Photonics K.K., Hamamatsu, Japan) was used to observe fluorescence.

Fluorescence Perfusion Pattern

The cholecystic arteries and veins were clearly visualized by excited fluorescence. Cholecystic veins were observed to flow in two directions, either extending directly into the gallbladder bed or into the hepatic hilum. The cholecystic artery appeared within 5 s of ICG injection, followed by the gallbladder wall and the cholecystic veins, constituting the 'gallbladder phase'. Following the gallbladder phase, the hepatic parenchyma appeared as a bright white light, persisting over a 10-min period of observation. Flow images varied in size from small to large, and in shape from round to segmental; this constituted the 'parenchymal phase'. We classified the fluorescence patterns during the parenchymal phase into two types according to the site and timing of fluorescence.

In type 1, the hepatic parenchyma adjacent to the gallbladder is stained immediately after the gallbladder phase, and the staining pattern coincides with the site receiving the cholecystic veins (fig. 1a). In type 2, the surfaces of liver segments distant

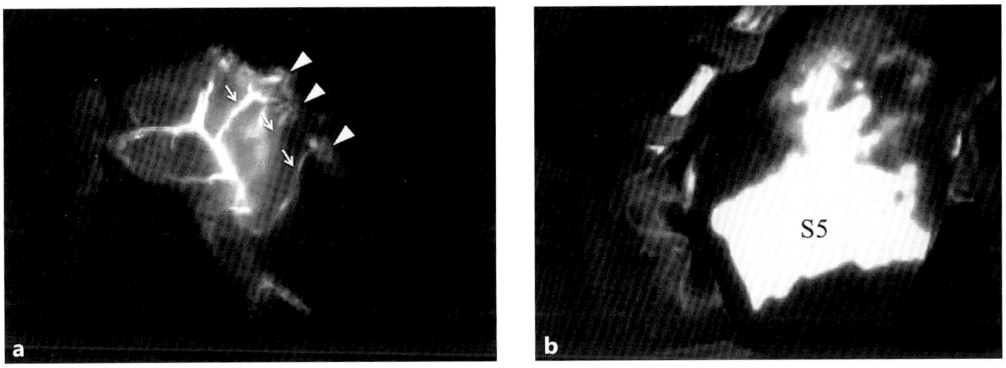

Fig. 1. a Fluorescence of the cholecystic veins (arrows). Fluorescence of the cholecystic veins flows directly into the hepatic parenchyma adjacent to the gallbladder (arrow heads). **b** Fluorescence is clearly identified in S5 (defined by Couinaud's nomenclature).

from the gallbladder stain in approximately 20–30 s after the gallbladder phase (fig. 1b). Type 1 sites appear during the early parenchymal phase, whereas type 2 sites appear over time. The two types then become mixed, and differentiation between them becomes impossible. It is important to differentiate between the two types of sites. One appears adjacent to the gallbladder and is relatively small in size; the other appears distant from the gallbladder and is larger in size with a segmental shape.

Cholecystic Venous Flow

Previous studies have addressed the cholecystic venous flow; Karlmark [13], Sappey [14] and Satoh [15] used cadaveric liver cast models created by injecting an artificial substance to evaluate this flow. Satoh described an association between the cholecystic veins and the intrahepatic portal branches; however, experiments using cast models may not accurately reflect the cholecystic dynamic blood flow in vivo.

Yoshimitsu et al. [16] performed CTA after superselective catheterization of the cholecystic artery and reported that the most frequent sites of cholecystic venous drainage around the gallbladder are S4 and S5. Sugita et al. [10] performed CTA in a similar manner and identified cholecystic veins flowing through the gallbladder bed into intrahepatic portal branches (P4a, P5) or hepatic sinusoids (S4a, S5). They termed the sinusoidal pooling of contrast material 'sinusoidal filling'. They were the first to notice a phenomenon in which the cholecystic veins flow directly into the hepatic parenchyma, identifying this as another route of cholecystic venous flow. Based on these findings, the cholecystic venous flow is thought to be one of the routes of hepatic metastasis in gallbladder carcinoma.

ICG fluorescence angiography has the advantage of detecting this blood flow in real time, and the procedure is quite sensitive; adequate fluorescence images are ob-

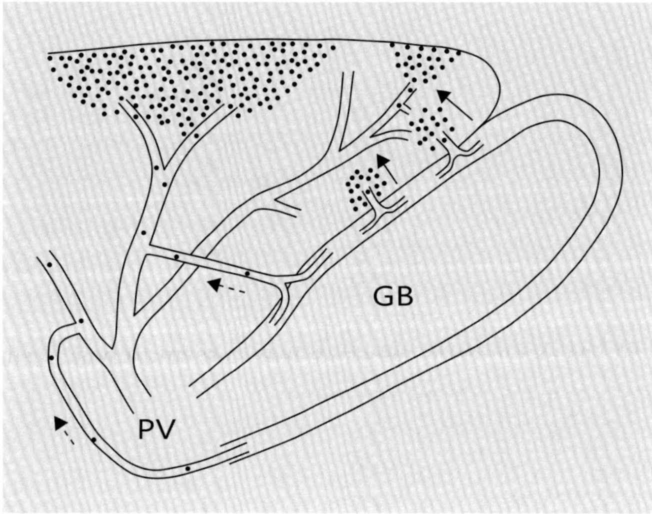

Fig. 2. Schematic representation of the hematogenous spread pattern. Type 1: the cholecystic vein flows directly into the hepatic parenchyma, occasionally reaching the peripheral intraportal branches (solid arrows). Type 2: the cholecystic vein flows into the intraportal branches (broken arrows). GB = Gallbladder; PV = Portal vein.

tained with small amounts of diluted ICG. However, this procedure does have some limitations. Only the blood flow at the surface of the liver may be observed because fluorescence located deep within the liver cannot be detected by the near-infrared camera system. Thus, connections between the cholecystic veins and the intraportal branches are not visualized. Nevertheless, the clinical simplicity and sensitivity of this technique are its great advantages. The PDE camera system can detect trace amounts of blood flow over time and is at least as sensitive as CTA. If not for this system, we could not have classified the cholecystic venous flow according to the site and timing of fluorescence.

The findings of various studies concerning the cholecystic venous flow can be reinterpreted through our study (fig. 2). In the present study, type 1 cholecystic venous flow proceeds directly into the hepatic parenchyma adjacent to the gallbladder. The sites demonstrate a bright white light immediately following the gallbladder phase. We speculate that this feature is probably similar to the sinusoidal filling seen on CTA by Sugita et al. [10]. In type 2 cholecystic venous flow, discrete sites of variable sizes and shapes appear at locations distant from the gallbladder (S4a, S5, and others) after the appearance of type 1 area, suggesting that a second cholecystic venous drainage route may be involved. The site and timing of fluorescence suggest that the cholecystic veins communicate with the intraportal branches, either through the hepatic hilum or through the gallbladder bed. The appearance of various shapes and sizes of fluorescence may be closely related to the venous communications with the intraportal branches; the more proximal the communication of the cholecystic vein, the broader the drainage area appears. Importantly, two thirds of our cases showed fluorescence in segments other than S4a or S5 [12]. We observed two different pathways of the cholecystic venous flow to the liver. Type 1 flows directly adjacent to the gallbladder, possibly corresponding to the site where angiolymphatic metastases have been observed [1, 2]; this may be the most likely site for hepatic metastases to occur. Our findings lead to the hypothesis that the type 1 pathway is the main route of hepatic metastasis and therefore plays a role in the localized hepatic metastases observed in early advanced gallbladder carcinoma.

Hepatic Resection for T2 Gallbladder Carcinoma

Based on the findings that the cholecystic veins flow into P4a and P5 [1, 15], anatomical S4a+S5 hepatic resection would seem to be a desirable procedure to ensure microscopic surgical margins. In a multicenter retrospective study, however, Araida et al. [17] found no significant difference in survival or recurrence rates between this anatomical resection and a more conventional extended cholecystectomy. Our study suggests that the cholecystic veins communicate not only with P4a and P5 but also with other intraportal branches because fluorescence is more widely distributed in the liver than would be expected based on the more limited communication theory. Therefore, it is not surprising that S4a+S5 hepatic resection does not show an advantage over conventional extended cholecystectomy.

The consensus is that extended cholecystectomy demonstrates better survival than simple cholecystectomy and that some hepatic resection is additionally required for T2 gallbladder carcinoma. Sufficient hepatic resection around the gallbladder bed, whether an anatomical S4a+S5 resection or a nonanatomical wedge resection, is needed to prevent recurrence, but defining the necessary extent of hepatic resection is controversial. We hypothesize that removing the liver parenchyma involved in type 1 flow is most important. Fluorescence angiography is currently considered the most effective way to evaluate this cholecystic venous flow.

We are currently using fluorescence angiography to perform hepatic resection according to each patient's individual cholecystic venous perfusion area. We consider the branch coursing to the gallbladder bed in the type 1 pathway to be the most important. Following the gallbladder phase, type 1 areas appear within S4a or S5. At this time, we mark the excited area on the liver surface by electrocautery. To remove liver parenchyma with an adequate margin, we perform hepatic resection 1 cm further than the edge of the marked area.

As mentioned above, the two types of fluorescence sites are sequentially identified. It is necessary to identify each type before they become mixed and impossible to differentiate. It is difficult, however, to correctly identify the type 1 area in a short period of time. We therefore visually confirm the course of cholecystic veins before ICG injection; cholecystic veins running on the surface of the gallbladder can be seen contacting the hepatic parenchyma adjacent to the gallbladder. Unfortunately, the cholecystic veins penetrating through the gallbladder bed are not detectable even with a near-infrared camera system. We can only confirm the presence of these penetrator veins by the appearance of excited areas on fluoroscopy.

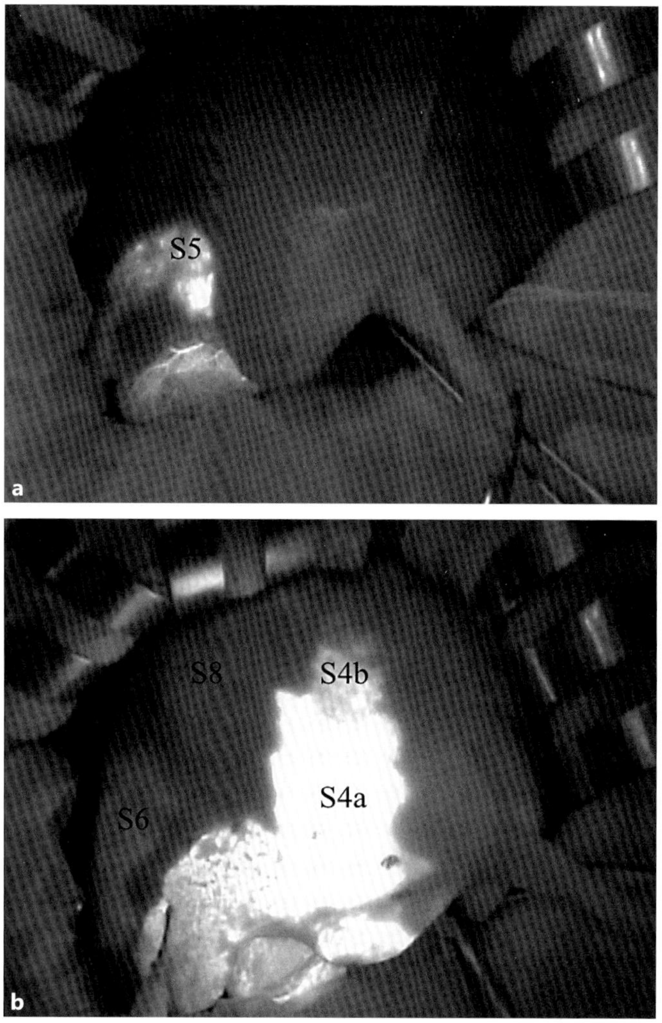

Fig. 3. a 15 s after the gallbladder phase, fluorescence is identified in S5 distant from the gallbladder; this is considered a type 1 area. **b** 45 s after the gallbladder phase, fluorescence is widely identified in S4a, S4b, S6 and S8; this is considered a type 2 area.

Since August 2008 we have performed surgical resection in 3 patients with gallbladder carcinoma suspected of subserosal invasion. In all patients, fluorescence angiography was used to determine the extent of hepatic resection. In one patient, discrete type 1 fluorescence appeared at a distance of 3 cm from the gallbladder (fig. 3a), and type 2 sites were subsequently identified in S4a, S4b and S6 (fig. 3b). We inferred that this type 1 fluorescence corresponded to the site in which the cholecystic penetrator veins flowed. Given these anatomic considerations, we selected a S4a+S5 hepatic resection to ensure a 1-cm disease-free margin. In the remaining 2 patients, we selected extended cholecystectomy. To date, all patients are recurrence-free.

In conclusion, fluorescence angiography makes it possible to clarify the site and extent of hepatectomy necessary for extended cholecystectomy. According to the cholecystic venous perfusion area, either an extended cholecystectomy or an S4a+S5 hepatic resection may be selected for each individual. The limitation in our study lies in the small number of patients and the consequent lack of statistical analysis. This procedure is based on the hypothesis that the type 1 pathway is the main route of hepatic metastasis in early advanced gallbladder carcinoma. To prove this hypothesis, we need to elucidate the role of the type 2 pathway. An association between the hepatic area involved in the type 2 pathway and the location of postoperative hepatic recurrence should be examined in the future.

References

1 Shirai Y, Tsukada K, Ohtani T, Watanabe H, Hatakeyama K: Hepatic metastases from carcinoma of the gallbladder. Cancer 1995;75:2063–2068.
2 Ohtsuka M, Miyazaki M, Itoh H, Nakagawa K, Ambiru S, Shimizu H, et al: Routes of hepatic metastasis of gallbladder carcinoma. Am J Clin Pathol 1998; 109:62–68.
3 Kondo S, Nimura Y, Kamiya J, Nagino M, Kanai M, Uesaka K, et al: Mode of tumor spread and surgical strategy in gallbladder carcinoma. Lagenbecks Arch Surg 2002;387:222–228.
4 Shimada H, Endo I, Fujii Y: Appraisal of surgical resection of gallbladder cancer with special reference to lymph node dissection. Lagenbecks Arch Surg 2000;385:509–514.
5 Wakai T, Shirai Y, Yokoyama N: Early gallbladder carcinoma does not warrant radical resection. Br J Surg 2001;88:675–678.
6 Paquet KJ: Appraisal of surgical resection of gallbladder carcinoma with special reference of hepatic resection. J Hepatobiliary Pancreat Surg 1998;5:299–2006.
7 Chijiiwa K, Nakano K, Ueda J, Noshiro H, Nagai E, Yamaguchi K, Tanaka M: Surgical treatment of patients with T2 gallbladder carcinoma invading the subserosal layer. J Am Coll Surg 2001;192:600–607.
8 Terazawa T, Miyake H, Kurahashi M, Tashiro S: Direct lymphatic spreading route into the liver from the gallbladder: an animal experiment using pig. J Med Invest 2004;51:210–217.
9 Yoshimitsu K, Honda H, Kuroiwa T, Irie H, Aibe H, Tajima T, et al: Liver metastasis from gallbladder carcinoma: anatomic correlation with cholecystic venous drainage demonstrated by helical computed tomography during injection of contrast medium in the cholecystic artery. Cancer 2001;92:340–348.
10 Sugita M, Ryu M, Satake M, Kinoshita T, Konishi M, Inoue K, et al: Intrahepatic inflow areas of the drainage vein of the gallbladder: analysis by angio-CT. Surgery 2001;128:417–421.
11 Ohtani Y, Wang Bai J, Poonkhum R, Ohtani O: Pathways for movement of fluid and cells from hepatic sinusoids to the portal lymphatic vessels and subcapsular region in rat livers. Arch Histol Cytol 2003;66: 239–252.
12 Kai K, Satoh S, Watanabe T, Endo Y: Evaluation of cholecystic venous flow using indocyanine green fluorescence angiography. J Hepatobiliary Pancreat Sci 2010;17:147–151.
13 Karlmark E: Die Localisationstendenz bei Venen in die Lever. Acta Pathol Microbiol Scand Suppl 1932; 13:100–119.
14 Sappey M: The anatomy of the veins of the gallbladder (quoted by Kreider PG). Surg Gynecol Obstet 1933;57:475–482.
15 Satoh T: Study of the anatomy of the venous drainage of the gallbladder (in Japanese). Tando 1989;3: 227–233.
16 Yoshimitsu K, Honda H, Kaneko K, Kuroiwa T, Irie H, Chijiiwa K, et al: Anatomy and clinical importance of cholecystic venous drainage: helical CT observations during injection of contrast medium into the cholecystic artery. AJR Am J Roentgenol 1997; 169:505–510.
17 Araida T, Higuchi R, Hamano M, Kodera Y, Takeshita N, Ota T, Yoshikawa T, Yamamoto M, Takasaki K: Hepatic resection in 485 R0 pT2 and pT3 cases of advanced carcinoma of the gallbladder: results of a Japanese Society of Biliary Surgery survey – a multicenter study. J Hepatobiliary Pancreato Sci 2009;16: 204–215.

Kyohei Kai
Department of Surgery, Japanese Red Cross Society Himeji Hospital
1-12-2 Shimoteno, Himeji
Hyogo 670-8540 (Japan)
E-Mail kai@hrc-hp.com

Kokudo N, Ishizawa T (eds): Fluorescent Imaging: Treatment of Hepatobiliary and Pancreatic Diseases.
Front Gastrointest Res. Basel, Karger, 2013, vol 31, pp 66–72 (DOI: 10.1159/000348612)

Fluorescence Cholangiography in Open Surgery

Noboru Mitsuhashi · Hiroaki Shimizu · Masaru Miyazaki

Department of General Surgery, Graduate School of Medicine, Chiba University, Chiba, Japan

Abstract

Although indocyanine green (ICG) fluorescence imaging has long been used in surgery for research purposes, its clinical use began relatively recently and is growing rapidly. ICG fluorescence imaging has advantages in that it: (1) enables the easy, rapid and real-time observation of internal organs using a safe agent, (2) has very high sensitivity, and (3) can identify pathological changes after repeated ICG administration. Therefore, it is widely used in many clinical departments for angiography, lymphangiography, sentinel lymph node visualization and tissue viability detection. The specificity of ICG kinetics makes it possible to acquire diverse information through its time-course distribution into the blood stream, liver parenchyma and biliary tract during abdominal surgery. Indeed, in biliary tract surgery the identification of arteries, veins and bile ducts by taking advantage of the transparency of biological tissues to infrared light, accurate identification of liver segments during intraportal ICG injection, its application in gallbladder cancer surgery based on the identification of the cystic vein perfusion area, utilization of its uptake in hepatocellular carcinoma and metastatic cancer in the liver, and high-sensitivity visualization of bile leakage during hepatectomy have been reported. In addition, ICG imaging has been performed during laparoscopy, making it a very useful technique in abdominal and laparoscopic surgeries. This technology is expected to be further utilized and advanced, and to contribute to clinical practice. This chapter describes the application of ICG fluorescence-based cholangiography to abdominal open surgery.

Fluorescence Cholangiography during Abdominal Surgery

Conventional X-ray-based cholangiography is very useful for the visualization of the biliary tree, which is often anomalous, and for the identification of iatrogenic intraoperative injury to the biliary tract, making it the most commonly used technique for cholangiography. However, it has disadvantages in that: (1) X-ray exposure is unavoidable, (2) roentgenoscopes are expensive and not versatile, (3) only bile duct images are obtained, and (4) the biliary tract needs to be punctured or incised during surgery. To offset these disadvantages, fluorescence cholangiography was developed, and a method using rolitetracycline and fluorescein was reported by Oddi et al. [1, 2] in 1996. In 2001, Holzinger et al. [3] visualized the biliary tree and bile leakage in rabbits by fluorescence cholangiography in laparotomy surgery. In 2006, Stiles et al. [4] reported the visualization of the biliary tree in mice by utilizing autofluorescence. In 2006, Kubota et al. [5] administered indocyanine green (ICG) intravenously to patients with liver transplantation and examined fluorescent bile to assess the blood flow in the hepatic artery and portal vein anastomosed using a SPY system (Novadeq Technologies). However, marked advances in this area started in 2006 when Hamamatsu Photonics developed and marketed the Photodynamic Eye (PDE) that was first reported by Kusano et al. [6] in Japan. Because of its relative inexpensiveness and wide range of applications, such as sentinel lymph node visualization and blood and lymph flow assessment, its use is growing explosively in the fields of brain, breast, gastrointestinal and cardiovascular surgery, dermatology, urology and obstetrics [7, 8]. In a pilot study conducted in 2008, we reported the first clinical case of ICG fluorescence cholangiography [9]. Later, a firm endoscope was developed which can be used for abdominal and laparoscopic surgeries. Therefore, ICG fluorescence cholangiography is expected to be more widely utilized [10, 11].

Detection Sensitivity of Indocyanine Green Fluorescence

ICG fluorescence cholangiography in abdominal surgery utilizes the fact that ICG, directly injected into the biliary tract, binds to blood proteins, is excreted into the bile and emits fluorescence on near-infrared irradiation. To begin with, we measured the sensitivity of ICG fluorescence using a PDE. Although ICG was previously considered to bind to serum albumin, it was reported to bind to α1-lipoprotein to emit fluorescence and was further shown to bind to high-density lipoprotein to emit a particularly strong fluorescence [12, 13]. To assess the sensitivity of ICG fluorescence using a PDE, we prepared tenfold serial dilutions of ICG (25 and 0.00025 μg/well in rows 1 and 6, respectively), to which physiological saline, bovine albumin, human serum or human bile was added, and determined the sensitively of ICG fluorescence using a conventional camera or a PDE (fig. 1a). The camera was able to detect the presence of ICG in the wells in rows 1 and 2. In contrast, the use of the PDE resulted in the emission of a fluorescence signal in mixtures with bovine albumin or human serum or bile, suggesting that ICG binds to various substances, such as albumin. The use of human serum resulted in the highest sensitivity, enabling the detection of fluorescence in the wells in rows 1–5. Although under conditions different from those in the human body, the sensitivity of ICG fluorescence was 100–1,000 times as high as that under visual examination.

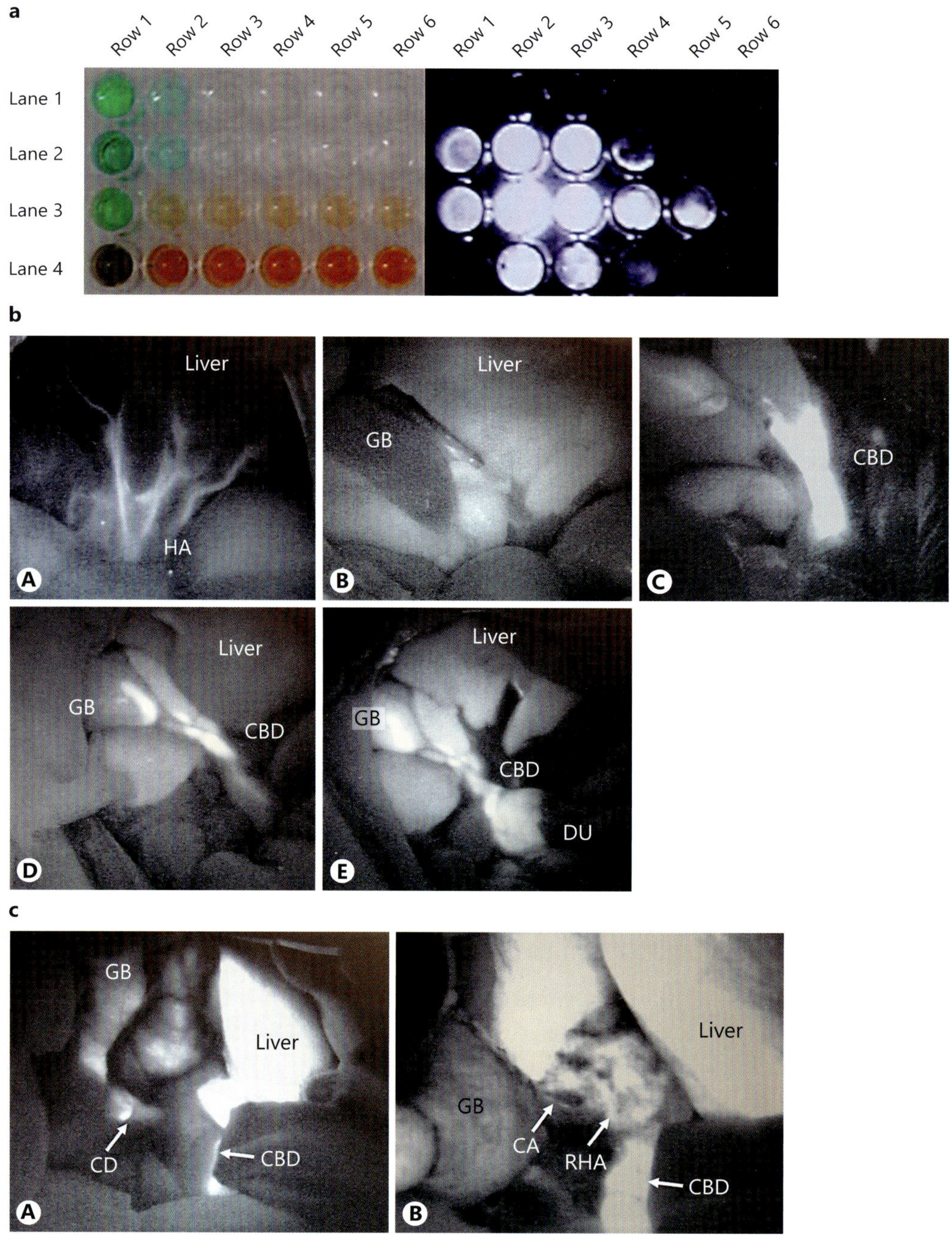

Fig. 1. a In vitro detection of ICG by infrared camera system. Left: normal camera; right: infrared camera. Lane 1: ICG alone; lane 2: ICG dissolved in 4 mg/ml bovine serum albumin; lane 3: ICG dissolved in human serum; lane 4: ICG dissolved in human bile juice. Row 1: ICG at 25 mg/well; row 2: ICG at 2.5 mg/well; row 3: ICG at 0.25 mg/well; row 4: ICG at 0.025 mg/well; row 5: ICG at 0.0025 mg/well; row 6: ICG at 0.00025 mg/well. Representative data are shown. **b** In vivo fluorescence detection over time in a pig. A: 10 s; B: 10 min; C: 20 min; D: 40 min; E: 60 min. HA = Hepatic artery; GB = gallbladder; CBD = common bile duct; DU = duodenum. **c** Fluorescence detection in a patient with cholecystectomy. A: Fluorescence at laparotomy; B: 10 s after additional ICG injection. CD = Cystic duct; CA = cystic artery. Reprinted from [9].

As described above, intraoperative cholangiography involves the direct injection of ICG into the biliary tract or the intravenous administration of ICG, which is excreted from hepatocytes into the bile and tested for fluorescence. Although the sensitivity of ICG fluorescence in bile when it was administered intravenously was not assessed, researchers reported the detection of a sufficiently high fluorescence signal [14–16]. As characteristically shown in the figure, ICG concentrations do not parallel the fluorescence signal intensity. The intensity of fluorescence is considered to be proportional to the concentration of the solute in the low range of concentrations, but reaches a saturation point beyond which a further increase in the solute concentration results in fluorescence quenching (i.e. fluorescence attenuation), which is ascribed to the self-absorption of fluorescence [17]. In this study, the ICG fluorescence in bovine albumin, human serum and human bile was significantly attenuated in the wells of row 1 compared to the wells in rows 2 and 3, apparently due to fluorescence quenching. ICG does not seem to have a low fluorescence emission due to fluorescence quenching unless a high concentration of ICG is directly mixed with bile. Generally, ICG is mixed with bile outside the body before its injection into the biliary tract; therefore, it is possible to detect the fluorescence emission and adjust the concentration of ICG at the time of mixture.

Time-Course Distribution of Indocyanine Green into the Blood Stream, Hepatocytes and Bile

We used minipigs to study the time-course distribution of ICG into the blood stream, hepatocytes and bile. The hepatic artery, liver, common bile duct, gallbladder and duodenum were visualized 10 s, 10 min, 20 min, 40 min and 60 min, respectively, after the injection of 0.5 ml of ICG (2.5 mg/ml) into the ear vein, indicating that the contrast effect varied according to the distribution of ICG (fig. 1b). We found that ICG fluorescence imaging enabled the observation of the time-dependent distribution of ICG with high sensitivity. Based on these results, we injected ICG 30 min before cholangiography in humans. However, in addition to species differences between humans and minipigs, the transfer of ICG from blood to bile depends on the hepatic blood flow and hepatocyte function. Therefore, the time required for radiography of the target site is considered to vary in patients undergoing surgery of the liver, many of whom have liver dysfunction due to hepatitis or cirrhosis, and the optimal time or dose of ICG administration remains unclear by our evaluation alone. However, various researchers reported that 2.5–12.5 mg/body of ICG was injected intravenously 30 min to 2 h before and during surgery, and a high level of fluorescence was observed in all cases [14–16]. The time required for the identification of the biliary tract naturally varies depending on the surgery involved. However, the biliary tract is visualized relatively early after ICG injection, the fluorescence remains in the biliary tract over a long period and the additional administration of ICG is simple; therefore, the intravenous injection of 2.5 mg of ICG seems to suffice.

Application of Indocyanine Green Fluorescence Cholangiography in Abdominal Surgery

For ICG fluorescence cholangiography, our patients undergoing open abdominal cholecystectomy received an intravenous injection of 2.5 mg of ICG 30 min before surgery and were examined for ICG fluorescence after laparotomy using a PDE (fig. 1c). The PDE main unit was covered with a sterile vinyl bag to avoid contamination of the surgical field, and PDE observations were performed at a distance of about 30 cm from the target. Since the shadowless light has an emitting wavelength in an infrared region similar to that of ICG at the time of fluorescence analysis and causes light interference, it needs to be switched off at the time of fluorescence analysis. However, this is not the case with ordinary fluorescent lights in the operating room. In our study, extrahepatic bile ducts were well visualized at the time of observation, and the cystic duct was also identifiable.

Various researchers have reported that the extrahepatic bile ducts and gallbladder can be very well visualized, posing no problems for the identification of normal biliary anatomy [14–16]. Although the biliary tree is often anomalous, a study reported that an accessory bile duct is identifiable, which contributes to performing a safer surgery. Ishizawa et al. [18] reported that although intravenously injected ICG is rapidly excreted into the bile, the sensitivity of ICG fluorescence cholangiography is so high that the fluorescence remains also in the liver parenchyma; therefore, it may be better to inject ICG into the biliary tract directly for hepatic operation. Furthermore, in patients undergoing cholecystectomy for an impacted stone in the cystic duct, only the upper side of the junction of the three bile ducts is visualized after intravenous injection; therefore, gallbladder puncture may be necessary for visualization, and the route of ICG administration should be determined for individual patients.

The transmission distance of infrared rays is several to 10 mm, and one should not visualize deep bile ducts or blood vessels and bile ducts that are covered with thick connective tissue and abundant adipose tissue. However, in patients with severe cholecystitis (which is not commonly encountered), it is very difficult to identify the course of the bile duct and cystic artery by inspection and palpation, but the ICG fluorescence method can confirm the presence or absence of vessels and bile ducts within the transmission distance of infrared rays, enabling us to perform a safer surgery. Thus, the ICG fluorescence method is expected to reduce intraoperative complications of open abdominal surgery and has been reported to show a significantly higher detection rate for bile leakage during hepatectomy than the routine leak test [19]. In addition, studies have reported the visualization of sentinel lymph nodes, assessment of blood flow, confirmation of organ viability in abdominal surgery, identification of blood vessels, liver segments, venous perfusion areas, visualization of bile leakage, assistance in surgery such as SILS (providing a poor surgical field), application to robotic surgery and visualization of choledocholithiasis [11, 20–22]. Ashitate et al. [23] reported fluorescence detection using a double-contrast technique with ICG and methylene blue, making the progress of intraoperative fluorescence cholangiography more promising.

A further increase in the number of reports on randomized control studies in clinical subjects is expected, and the significance of the ICG fluorescence method will be established. As gastrointestinal endoscopy with narrow band imaging has become the standard method, the ICG fluorescence method may become indispensable. Thus, the ICG fluorescence method will definitely become a breakthrough in abdominal surgery.

Conclusions

ICG fluorescence imaging has advantages in that it: (1) enables the easy, rapid and real-time observation of internal organs using a relatively inexpensive equipment, (2) has very high sensitivity, and (3) can identify pathological changes after repeated ICG administration. Along with laparoscopic ICG fluorescence imaging, this imaging technique is expected to find more clinical applications.

References

1 Oddi A, Mills CO, Custureri F, Di Nicola V, Elias E, Di Matteo G: Intraoperative biliary tree imaging with cholyl-lysyl-fluorescein: an experimental study in the rabbit. Surg Laparosc Endosc 1996;6:198–200.

2 Oddi A, Di Nicola V, Panzini A, Berni A, Lucci S, Greco L, Urciuoli P, Custureri F: The intraoperative visualization of the bile ducts by the use of fluorescent substances. A feasibility study. G Chir 1996;17:620–623.

3 Holzinger F, Krähenbühl L, Schteingart CD, Ton-Nu HT, Hofmann AF: Use of a fluorescent bile acid to enhance visualization of the biliary tract and bile leaks during laparoscopic surgery in rabbits. Surg Endosc 2001;15:209–212.

4 Stiles BM, Adusumilli PS, Bhargava A, Fong Y: Fluorescent cholangiography in a mouse model: an innovative method for improved laparoscopic identification of the biliary anatomy. Surg Endosc 2006;20: 1291–1295.

5 Kubota K, Kita J, Shimoda M, Rokkaku K, Kato M, Iso Y, Sawada T: Intraoperative assessment of reconstructed vessels in living-donor liver transplantation, using a novel fluorescence imaging technique. J Hepatobiliary Pancreat Surg 2006;13:100–104.

6 Kusano M, Kato M, Nakao K, Shimizu Y, Tajima Y, Yamazaki K, Aoki T, Kaetsu T, Tsunoda A, Miwa M: A novel method of the detection of sentinel node by the LED emission ICG fluorescence in gastrointestinal cancers. Japan Soc Gastroenterol Surg 2006;39: 1464.

7 Gioux S, Choi HS, Frangioni JV: Image-guided surgery using invisible near-infrared light: fundamentals of clinical translation. Mol Imaging 2010;9:237–255.

8 Tagaya N, Aoyagi H, Nakagawa A, Abe A, Iwasaki Y, Tachibana M, Kubota K: A novel approach for sentinel lymph node identification using fluorescence imaging and image overlay navigation surgery in patients with breast cancer. World J Surg 2011;35:154–158.

9 Mitsuhashi N, Kimura F, Shimizu H, Imamaki M, Yoshidome H, Ohtsuka M, Kato A, Yoshitomi H, Nozawa S, Furukawa K, Takeuchi D, Takayashiki T, Suda K, Igarashi T, Miyazaki M: Usefulness of intraoperative fluorescence imaging to evaluate local anatomy in hepatobiliary surgery. J Hepatobiliary Pancreat Surg 2008;15:508–514.

10 Ishizawa T, Bandai Y, Ijichi M, Kaneko J, Hasegawa K, Kokudo N: Fluorescent cholangiography illuminating the biliary tree during laparoscopic cholecystectomy. Br J Surg 2010;97:1369–1377.

11 Buchs NC, Hagen ME, Pugin F, Volonte F, Bucher P, Schiffer E, Morel P: Intra-operative fluorescent cholangiography using indocyanin green during robotic single site cholecystectomy. Int J Med Robot 2012;8: 436–440.

12 Baker KJ: Binding of sulfobromophthalein (BSP) sodium and indocyanine green (ICG) by plasma alpha-1 lipoproteins. Proc Soc Exp Biol Med 1966;122: 957–963.

13 Yoneya S, Saito T, Komatsu Y, Koyama I, Takahashi K, Duvoll-Young J: Binding properties of indocyanine green in human blood. Invest Ophthalmol Vis Sci 1998;39:1286–1290.
14 Ishizawa T, Bandai Y, Ijichi M, Kaneko J, Hasegawa K, Kokudo N: Fluorescent cholangiography illuminating the biliary tree during laparoscopic cholecystectomy. Br J Surg 2010;97:1369–1377.
15 Aoki T, Murakami M, Yasuda D, Shimizu Y, Kusano T, Matsuda K, Niiya T, Kato H, Murai N, Otsuka K, Kusano M, Kato T: Intraoperative fluorescent imaging using indocyanine green for liver mapping and cholangiography. J Hepatobiliary Pancreat Sci 2010; 17:590–594.
16 Tagaya N, Shimoda M, Kato M, Nakagawa A, Abe A, Iwasaki Y, Oishi H, Shirotani N, Kubota K: Intraoperative exploration of biliary anatomy using fluorescence imaging of indocyanine green in experimental and clinical cholecystectomies. J Hepatobiliary Pancreat Sci 2010;17:595–600.
17 Benson RC, Kues HA: Fluorescence properties of indocyanine green as related to angiography. Phys Med Biol 1978;23:159–163.
18 Ishizawa T, Tamura S, Masuda K, Aoki T, Hasegawa K, Imamura H, Beck Y, Kokudo N: Intraoperative fluorescent cholangiography using indocyanine green: a biliary road map for safe surgery. J Am Coll Surg 2009;208:e1–e4.
19 Kaibori M, Ishizaki M, Matsui K, Kwon AH: Intraoperative indocyanine green fluorescent imaging for prevention of bile leakage after hepatic resection. Surgery 2011;150:91–98.
20 Ishizawa T, Kaneko J, Inoue Y, Takemura N, Seyama Y, Aoki T, Beck Y, Sugawara Y, Hasegawa K, Harada N, Ijichi M, Kusaka K, Shibasaki M, Bandai Y, Kokudo N: Application of fluorescent cholangiography to single-incision laparoscopic cholecystectomy. Surg Endosc 2011;25:2631–2636.
21 Figueiredo JL, Siegel C, Nahrendorf M, Weissleder R: Intraoperative near-infrared fluorescent cholangiography (NIRFC) in mouse models of bile duct injury. World J Surg 2010;34:336–343.
22 Verbeek FP, van der Vorst JR, Schaafsma BE, Hutteman M, Bonsing BA, van Leeuwen FW, Frangioni JV, van de Velde CJ, Swijnenburg RJ, Vahrmeijer AL: Image-guided hepatopancreatobiliary surgery using near-infrared fluorescent light. J Hepatobiliary Pancreat Sci 2012;19:626–637.
23 Ashitate Y, Stockdale A, Choi HS, Laurence RG, Frangioni JV: Real-time simultaneous near-infrared fluorescence imaging of bile duct and arterial anatomy. J Surg Res 2012;176:7–13.

Noboru Mitsuhashi
Department of General Surgery
Graduate School of Medicine, Chiba University
1-8-1 Inohana, Chuo-ku, Chiba 260-0856 (Japan)
E-Mail noborumitsuhashi@gmail.com

Kokudo N, Ishizawa T (eds): Fluorescent Imaging: Treatment of Hepatobiliary and Pancreatic Diseases.
Front Gastrointest Res. Basel, Karger, 2013, vol 31, pp 73–79 (DOI: 10.1159/000348615)

Fluorescence Cholangiography in Laparoscopic Cholecystectomy: Experience in Japan

Nobumi Tagaya · Yoshitake Sugamata · Nana Makino · Kazuyuki Saito · Takashi Okuyama · Shinichiro Koketsu · Masatoshi Oya

Department of Surgery, Dokkyo Medical University Koshigaya Hospital, Koshigaya, Japan

Abstract

We describe a new modality for intraoperative exploration of the biliary anatomy using fluorescence imaging with indocyanine green (ICG) and its evaluation in 15 patients diagnosed as having gallbladder stones who were scheduled to undergo laparoscopic cholecystectomy. The patients included 6 males and 9 females with a mean age of 54 years and a mean BMI of 22.3. Standard four-port laparoscopic cholecystectomy was performed in 11 patients and single-incision laparoscopic cholecystectomy in the other 4. ICG was infused 1 h before surgery. We observed the biliary tract under real-time fluorescence imaging guidance, and confirmed the positions of the gallbladder, cystic duct, and common bile and hepatic duct on the monitor. The cystic artery was also observed after reinjection of ICG. The procedure was completed successfully in all cases, and no additional ports or conversion to open cholecystectomy were necessary. The mean operation time was 88 min. We obtained a clear view of the biliary tract in all patients, and the cystic artery was confirmed 10 s after reinjection of ICG. There were no specific perioperative complications related to the intravenous injection of ICG. The median postoperative hospital stay was 3 days. Intraoperative exploration of the biliary tract using ICG is a useful approach for identification of the biliary anatomy without cannulation into the cystic duct, X-ray equipment or use of radioactive materials. We expect that this modality will become routine, offering a lower degree of invasiveness that will help avoid bile duct injury.

Cholecystectomy is a surgical technique that has become standardized worldwide. Although laparoscopic cholecystectomy became possible in the early 1990s, this was initially associated with an increase in the incidence of bile duct injury (BDI) from

0.2 to 0.5% [1], and a recent study revealed that such BDI had a significant negative impact on quality of life even 10 years after the event [2]. The primary cause of BDI is an error of visual perception in 71–97% of cases, not insufficient technical skill of the surgeon [3, 4]. Factors that impede visual assessment and increase the risk of BDI include previous or ongoing inflammation, variant ductal anatomy, and limited surgical experience [1, 5]. To prevent BDI, there are several different modalities for intraoperative assessment of the biliary anatomy during cholecystectomy [6]. Here we introduce a new method for intraoperative exploration of the biliary anatomy using fluorescence imaging with indocyanine green (ICG) (Diagnogreen; Daiichi Sankyo Co., Tokyo, Japan) and evaluates its clinical utility for laparoscopic cholecystectomy.

Materials and Methods

This study included 15 patients diagnosed as having gallbladder stones, who had laparoscopic cholecystectomy planned between May 2009 and September 2011. There were 6 males and 9 females, ranging in age from 37 to 69 years (mean: 54), and with a BMI of 19.5–27.3 (mean 22.3). Standard four-port laparoscopic cholecystectomy was performed in 11 patients and single-incision laparoscopic cholecystectomy in the other 4. ICG (1.0 ml/body of 2.5 mg/ml ICG) was injected 1 h before the initial skin incision at surgery. The study was approved by the ethics committees of Dokkyo Medical University and Dokkyo Medical University Koshigaya Hospital. Informed consent was obtained from all patients.

Laparoscopic Approach
With the patient under general anesthesia, we created four ports (a 12-mm port at the center of the midline, and three 5-mm ports in the subxiphoid and right subcostal regions) or a 2.5-cm skin incision at the umbilicus with a surgical glove (size: 5.5) containing three 5-mm ports attached to a wound retractor in the peritoneal cavity after creating pneumoperitoneum by CO_2 insufflation or an abdominal wall-lifting method. Using a laparoscope with infrared function (Olympus K.K., Tokyo, Japan; Hamamatsu Photonics, Hamamatsu, Japan; Shinko Optical, Tokyo, Japan), we observed the area from the hepatic hilum to the duodenum at the point of initial insertion of the laparoscope under fluorescence imaging guidance during the division (fig. 1), after identification and dissection of the cystic duct and artery (fig. 2), and before closure of the wounds, respectively. To observe blood flow within the cystic artery, ICG (2.5 mg/ml) was re-administered intravenously through the venous line after identifying the vessel structure. If the florescence image was unclear due to inflammation around the gallbladder or dense adipose tissue in the hepatoduodenal ligament, an originally manufactured transparent flat plastic device was used to achieve local compression, allowing clearer fluorescence imaging over the biliary tract.

Results

No conversions to open cholecystectomy were necessary. The operation time ranged from 68 to 118 min, with a mean of 88 min. The estimated blood loss was minimal and we were able to clearly visualize the biliary tract in all patients. The cystic duct,

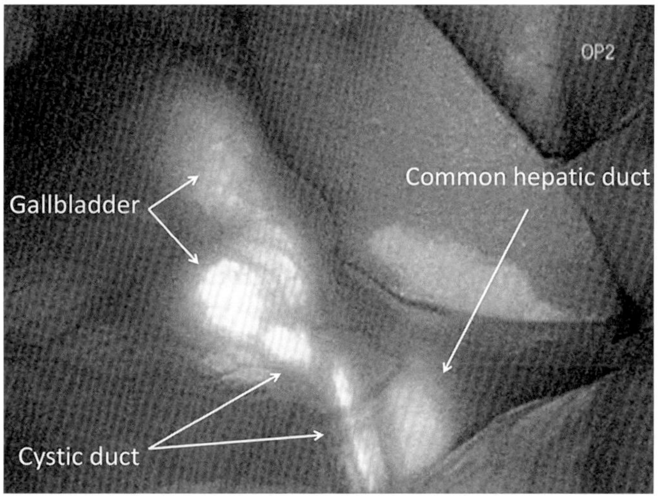

Fig. 1. Fluorescence image obtained at the time of initial insertion of the laparoscope.

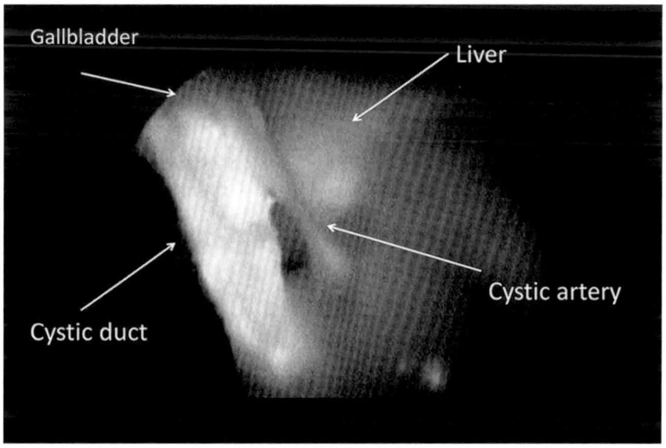

Fig. 2. Fluorescence image after identification of the cystic duct and artery.

common bile duct and common hepatic duct were identified via the laparoscope. The gallbladder was not clearly visualized by fluorescence imaging due to inflammation or an impacted stone in the gallbladder neck. Local compression with our transparent plastic device provided a clearer view of the biliary tract. In particular, the confluence of the cystic duct and the common bile duct was adequately identified. Although the location of and blood flow within the cystic artery were not easily confirmed via the laparoscope in the first few cases, they were clearly identified approximately 10 s after reinjection of ICG as the surgeons gained experience. There were no adverse events related to the intraoperative procedure itself or the use of ICG. The mean postoperative hospital stay was 3 days, and there were no postoperative complications.

Discussion

Several methods for intraoperative assessments and identification of the biliary anatomy during surgery are available when performing cholecystectomy. They are intended to allow road mapping for a safe surgical procedure and prevention of BDI. Such assessments include intraoperative cholangiography via cannulation of the cystic duct [7, 8], laparoscopic ultrasound [9, 10], cholecystocholangiography [11], drip infusion cholangiography [12], dye cholangiography [13], light cholangiography [14] or near-infrared cholangiography [15–19] in clinical studies, and passive infrared cholangiography [20] or hyperspectral cholangiography [21] in animal studies. Each has its advantages and disadvantages in terms of applicability, the findings afforded, safety, ease of use, time required, etc. Although near-infrared fluorescence cholangiography is still at an early stage of development relative to established intraoperative cholangiography, it may be superior to other modalities in terms of real-time observation, noninvasiveness and ease of performance.

ICG becomes stabilized in serum after intravenous injection, and has a peak fluorescence wavelength of 845 nm when exposed to near-infrared radiation with a wavelength of 760 nm. ICG is known to be safe at the doses used in routine clinical procedures, and particularly for evaluation of liver function. ICG is administered at only 1 ml/body (0.04–0.05 mg/kg) at a concentration of 2.5 mg/ml for intraoperative exploration of the biliary tract. Recently, its characteristics have been exploited for identification of sentinel lymph nodes in patients with breast [22] or gastrointestinal [23] cancer. However, there have been few clinical reports on the use of ICG fluorescence imaging of the biliary tract, and its usefulness is still not widely recognized.

The timing of ICG injection is an important consideration for better fluorescence imaging. Several reports have indicated that it should be performed 30 min before surgery [15], 30–45 min before surgery with a second injection approximately 45 min after the first if fluorescence is not detected in the liver [19], or after endotracheal intubation of the patient in the operating room [18]. We have routinely injected ICG 1 h before surgery, resulting in a minimal shine-through effect from the liver, and consider this timing to be optimal for fluorescence imaging of the hepatobiliary system [17].

As the depth of penetration of infrared light through tissue is limited to only 3–5 mm [15] or 5–10 mm [24], tissue thickness strongly affects the intensity of fluorescence. In cholecystectomy, the thickness of the gallbladder wall or its adjacent connective tissues is affected by obesity or edema and dense adhesion due to acute or chronic inflammation. Buchs et al. [19] reported that fluorescence images of the cystic, common and hepatic ducts were recognizable before dissection of Calot's triangle in 91.7, 50 and 33.3% of patients compared with 100, 83.3 and 66.7%, respectively, after dissection. Therefore, to improve identification of the biliary tree by fluorescence imaging, we applied an originally manufactured transparent flat plastic device [17].

This allowed us to recognize the fluorescence images of the cystic, common bile and hepatic ducts before dissection in all patients. This device increased the intensity of fluorescence from the biliary tract by compression at local points, and we think that it is useful for preventing BDI in complicated cases.

The advantages of this method are that it requires no cannulation into the cystic duct, no special arrangements for X-ray equipment and no exposure to radioactivity. Fluorescence imaging can be easily obtained by switching to the infrared camera via a hand- or foot-operated device without any preparation for an additional procedure. The location of blood vessels around the cystic duct can be visualized repeatedly by reinfusion of ICG. This method is very useful for exploration of biliary anatomy without the risk of bile duct and blood vessel injury. Anatomical anomalies of the bile duct or hepatic artery are often encountered during hepatobiliary surgery. Ishizawa et al. [18] reported that an accessory bile duct was detected in 100% of cases by fluorescence cholangiography after dissection of Calot's triangle, compared with 75% when employing intraoperative drip infusion cholangiography. Although fluorescence imaging may not clearly demonstrate such biliary anomalies before dissection of Calot's triangle, application of the transparent flat plastic device can dramatically improve the rate of detection of biliary tree fluorescence. Furthermore, the location of the hepatic artery or its branches can be recognized in real time by reinfusion of ICG during the procedure. Furthermore, near-infrared endoscopy has high sensitivity for bile juice, allows early recognition of bile leakage, facilitates early treatment and thus minimizes bile duct injury. In fact, when we performed ordinary intraoperative cholangiography after fluorescence imaging, we easily recognized leakage of fluorescent bile juice from the small orifice in the cystic duct created for insertion of the cannula [17]. In terms of detection of minimal bile juice leakage, fluorescence imaging is absolutely superior to the image obtained on an ordinary two-dimensional monitor during laparoscopic cholecystectomy.

Currently, there are several issues that need to be considered when performing intraoperative assessment of the biliary anatomy. Firstly, to allow easy identification under fluorescence imaging, another reagent yielding a high intensity of fluorescence, or a near-infrared fluorophore such as the carboxylic acid form of IRDye™ 800 CW (CW800-CA), would be preferable as it is very difficult to achieve sufficient identification of the biliary anatomy under ICG guidance in the presence of dense connective tissues or thickening due to inflammation. However, due to a variety of intellectual property, regulatory and commercial issues beyond the control of academic investigations, the above reagent is unlikely to become clinically available for at least another 5–10 years [25]. Secondly, although ordinary intraoperative cholangiography can detect stones in the common bile duct as defects, our experience suggests that this method still leaves a degree of uncertainty regarding the recognition of common bile duct stones. In fact, even with open cholecystectomy we were unable to detect common bile duct stones that had been diagnosed before surgery using fluorescence imaging. The presence of fluorescing bile around stones in the common bile duct may mask the stones themselves [18]. Therefore, preoperative evaluation using interventional radiology is still mandatory for the treatment of stones in the common bile duct. Further studies are needed to address these issues.

In conclusion, intraoperative exploration of the biliary tract using ICG is a useful navigation modality for identification of the biliary anatomy without the need for cannulation into the cystic duct, X-ray equipment or use of radioactive materials, and manipulation with the left hand using ordinary laparoscopic instruments is a necessary skill to acquire in order to achieve successful and safe single-incision laparoscopic cholecystectomy. We expect that this method will become routine, offering a lower degree of invasiveness that will help avoid bile duct injury.

References

1 Nuzzo G, Giuliante F, Giovannini I, Ardito F, D'Acapito F, Vellone M, Murazio M, Capelli G: Bile duct injury during laparoscopic cholecystectomy: results of an Italian national survey on 56,591 cholecystectomies. Arch Surg 2005;140:986–992.

2 De Reuver PR, Sprangers MA, Rauws EA, Lameris JS, Busch OR, van Gulik TM, Gouma DJ: Impact of bile duct injury after laparoscopic cholecystectomy on quality of life: a longitudinal study after multidisciplinary treatment. Endoscopy 2008;40:837–643.

3 Way LW Stewart L, Gantert W, Liu K, Lee CM, Whang K, Hunter JG: Causes and prevention of laparoscopic bile duct injuries: analysis of 252 cases from a human factors and cognitive psychology perspective. Ann Surg 2003;237:450–469.

4 Olsen D: Bile duct injuries during laparoscopic cholecystectomy. Surg Endosc 1997;11:133–138.

5 Meyers WC, Peterseim DS, Pappas TN, Schauer PR, Eubanks S, Murray E, Suhocki P: Low insertion of hepatic segmental duct VII-VIII is an important cause of major biliary injury or misdiagnosis. Am J Surg 1996;171:187–191.

6 Buddingh KT, Nieuwenhuijs VB, van Buuren L, Hulscher JBF, De Jong JS, van Dam GM: Intraoperative assessment of biliary anatomy for prevention of bile duct injury: a review of current and future patient safety interventions. Surg Endosc 2011;25: 2449–2461.

7 Waade A, Nilsson M: Iatrogenic bile duct injury: a population-based study of 152,776 cholecystectomies in the Swedish Inpatient Registry. Arch Surg 2006;141:1207–1213.

8 Giger U, Ouaissi M, Schmitz SF, Krahenbuhl S, Krahenbuhl I: Bile duct injury and use of cholangiography during laparoscopic cholecystectomy. Br J Surg 2011;98:391–396.

9 Biffl WL, Moore EE, Offner PJ, Francinose RJ, Bruch JM: Routine intraoperative laparoscopic ultrasonography with selective cholangiography reduces bile duct complications during laparoscopic cholecystectomy. J Am Coll Surg 2001;193:272–280.

10 Machi J, Johnson JO, Deziel DJ, Soper NJ, Berber E, Siperstein A, Hata M, Patel S, Singh K, Arregui ME: The routine use of laparoscopic ultrasound decreases bile duct injury: a multicenter study. Surg Endosc 2009;23:384–388.

11 Daoud M, McCallum MJ: An easy and effective method of cholangiography in laparoscopic cholecystectomy: laparoscopic cholecystocholangiography. Aust NZ J Surg 1999;69:138–140.

12 Ochiai T, Yamazaki S, Ohta K, Takahashi M, Iwai T, Irie T, Noguchi N, Takamatsu S, Kawamura T, Teramoto K, Arii S: Is drip infusion cholangiography (DIC) an acceptable modality at cholecystectomy for cholecystolithasis, considering the frequency of bile duct maljunction and intraoperative bile duct injury? J Hepatobiliary Pancreat Surg 2004;11:135–139.

13 Sari YS, Tunali V, Tomaoglu K, Karagoz B, Guneyi A, Karagoz I: Can bile duct injury be prevented? A new technique in laparoscopic cholecystectomy. BMC Surg 2005;5:14.

14 Xu F, Xu CG, Xu DZ: A new method of preventing bile duct injury in laparoscopic cholecystectomy. World J Gastroenterol 2004;10:2916–2918.

15 Mitsuhashi N, Kimura F, Shimizu H, Imamaki M, Yoshidome H, Ohtsuka M, Kato A, Yoshitomi H, Nozawa S, Furukawa K, Takeuchi D, Takayashiki T, Suda K, Igarashi T, Miyazaki M: Usefulness of intraoperative fluorescence imaging to evaluate local anatomy in hepatobiliary surgery. J Hepatobilary Pancreat Surg 2008;15:508–514.

16 Aoki T, Murakami M, Yasuda D, Shimizu Y, Kusano T, Matsuda K, Niiya T, Kato H, Murai N, Otsuka K, Kusano M, Kato T: Intraoperative fluorescent imaging using indocyanine green for liver mapping and cholangiography. J Hepatobiliary Pancreat Sci 2012; 17:590–594.
17 Tagaya N, Shimoda M, Kato M, Nakagawa A, Abe A, Iwasaki Y, Oishi H, Shirotani N, Kubota K: Intraoperative exploration of biliary anatomy using fluorescence imaging of indocyanine green in experimental and clinical cholecystectomies. J Hepatobiliary Pancreat Sci 2010;17:595–600.
18 Ishizawa T, Bandai Y, Ijichi M, Kaneko J, Hasegawa K, Kokudo N: Fluorescent cholangiography illuminating the biliary tree during laparoscopic cholecystectomy. Br J Surg 2010;97:1369–1377.
19 Buchs NC, Hagen ME, Pugin F, Volonte F, Bucher P, Schiffer E, Morel P: Intra-operative fluorescent cholangiography using indocyanine green during robotic single site cholecystectomy. Int J Med Robotics Comput Assist Surg 2012;8:436–440.
20 Liu JJ, Alemozaffar M, NcHone B, Dhanani N, Gage F, Pinto PA, Gorback AM, Elster E: Evaluation of real-time infrared intraoperative cholangiography in a porcine model. Surg Endosc 2008;22:2659–2664.
21 Livinston EH, Gulaka P, Kommera S, Wang B, Liu H: In vivo spectroscopic characterization of porcine biliary tract tissues: first step in the development of new biliary tract imaging devices. Ann Biomed Eng 2009; 37:201–209.
22 Tagaya N, Yamazaki R, Nakagawa A, Abe A, Hamada K, Kubota K, Oyama T: Intraoperative identification of sentinel lymph nodes by near-infrared fluorescence imaging in patients with breast cancer. Am J Surg 2008;195:850–853.
23 Kusano M, Tajima Y, Yamazaki K, Kato M, Watanabe M, Miwa M: Sentinel node mapping guided by indocyanine green fluorescence imaging: a new method for sentinel node navigation surgery in gastrointestinal cancer. Dig Surg 2008;25:103–108.
24 Kim SA, Lim YT, Soltesz EG, Grand AM, Lee J, Nakayama A, et al: Near-infrared fluorescent type II quantum dots for sentinel lymph node mapping. Nat Biotechnol 2004;22:93–97.
25 Matsui A, Tanaka E, Choi HS, Winer JH, Kianzad V, Gioux S, Laurence RG, Frangioni JV: Real-time intraoperative near-infrared fluorescence identification of the extrahepatic bile ducts using clinically available contrast agents. Surgery 2010;148:87–95.

Nobumi Tagaya
Department of Surgery, Dokkyo Medical University Koshigaya Hospital
2-1-50 Minamikoshigaya
Koshigaya, Saitama 343-8555 (Japan)
E-Mail tagaya@dokkyomed.ac.jp

Kokudo N, Ishizawa T (eds): Fluorescent Imaging: Treatment of Hepatobiliary and Pancreatic Diseases.
Front Gastrointest Res. Basel, Karger, 2013, vol 31, pp 80–85 (DOI: 10.1159/000348621)

Fluorescence Cholangiography in Laparoscopic Cholecystectomy Experience in Argentina

Fernando D. Dip · Mario Nahmod · Lisandro Alle · Luis Sarotto · Francisco Suarez Anzorena · Pedro Ferraina

Department of Surgery, Hospital de Clinicas "José de San Martín", University of Buenos Aires, Buenos Aires, Argentina

Abstract

The frequency of laparoscopic cholecystectomies in Argentina has increased in the last few years. The use of intraoperative methods for the detection of bile ducts such as intraoperative cholangiography (IOC) varies within the country although it is a routine procedure in our workplace. Surgical injuries in bile ducts remain a constant, amounting to about 0.4%. This is the reason why we have been looking for an easy alternative to IOC, with the aim to reduce those numbers. Sponsored by the company Karl Storz, in 2011 we started performing fluorescence cholangiography in our laparoscopic cholecystectomies; we have kept those records prospectively and now have a total of 65 cases. The use of this method seems promising with some clear advantages such as its low cost, real-time performance and the possibility to visualize structures before they are sectioned. We have been able to visualize the main bile duct without dissection in 89.5% of the cases. Areas that still need improvement include some technical issues such as the depth for visualization in obese patients or in those with severe or substantially chronic inflammatory stages where the light cannot penetrate tissues appropriately.

When laparoscopic surgery started at the beginning of the 1990s, surgical techniques were modified. After the initial learning curve within groups specialized in hepatobiliary-pancreatic surgery, it became evident that the frequency of injury to the bile duct increased by 100%, i.e. 0.2–0.4% more serious injuries with sections and resections of the main bile duct which in some cases included the two hepatic ducts by the hilar plate and the hepatic artery [1].

The difficulty of locating the bile duct intraoperatively and the challenge of laparoscopy with flat vision increases the difficulty of recognizing the precise anatomy of the bile duct. If we take into account that anatomic variations are very frequent, the best way to prevent injuries is to locate Calot's triangle, composed of the bile duct, cystic duct and liver, within which the cystic artery is found. To diminish the rate of surgical injuries to the bile duct, technical resources such as Strasberg's critical view of safety, Grossman's triangle dissection and the use of intraoperative cholangiography (IOC) became common practice.

The History of Intraoperative Cholangiography

The first IOC was performed by the Argentinian surgeon and professor Dr. Pablo Luis Mirizzi in the province of Córdoba in the Argentine Republic on June 18, 1931 [2]. The patient suffered from gallbladder hydrops and the IOC showed a normal bile duct. The source of inspiration for Dr. Mirizzi was the work of Carnot and Blamoutier in 1921 in which a barium mixture was injected postoperatively through an external bile fistula showing the characteristics of the bile duct. Mirizzi and his cholangiography undoubtedly mark a turning point in biliary surgery. The procedure was quickly adopted and after a long period during which nobody had argued its systematic use, there was some questioning, after which it was prescribed selectively [3–6].

The Importance of Radioscopic Cholangiography in Cholecystectomy
IOC allows for the diagnosis of variations in the anatomy of the bile duct in 6–10%, such as the opening of the cystic duct into the right hepatic duct, the low joint of both hepatic ducts, or the isolated and low opening of the posterior right collecting duct [7]. The latter may be present in up to 20% of cases and its importance rests in the fact that this is the only one located outside the liver among the different variations of the proximal bile confluence and it is a factor that may lead to its injury when the dissection of the gallbladder site becomes difficult and has to be done deeply towards the hepatic parenchyma [3].

The IOC is used to assess the intra- and extrahepatic anatomy of the bile duct, anatomic variations, and VBP caliper, as well as detect VBP calculi. Although most centers use this method 'systematically', some groups use it 'selectively' in case VBP lithiasis is suspected or to confirm its anatomy when in doubt [8]. Nevertheless, one of the problems that IOC has not solved is that in order to perform it it is necessary to section. One way or another, if the duct which was sectioned is the right hepatic duct or the choledochus, the surgical injury of the bile duct has already been caused.

Radioscopic cholangiography has some downsides such as increased cost, the use of radiation and increased operative time. The current situation in Argentina is that the presence of imaging equipment in the operation theater for each laparoscopic cholecystectomy is not homogeneous. In many cases in fact, the decision to use such equipment to perform a radioscopic cholangiography is made by the surgeon according to their experience or when an injury is suspected.

Facing a problem which has yet to be solved, we have started to research real-time methods which require no sectioning of any structures for identification [9]. This is why we have started to implement fluorescence as an identification method of the biliary structures with the use of a dye and a specific source of light.

Experience in Argentina

The aim of our study was to demonstrate the identification of the different biliary structures, making use of a new cholangiographic technique in real time and without modifying the laparoscopic view by using a fluorescent dye injected intravenously that can be visualized with infrared light.

Materials and Methods

The study was approved by the ethics committees of the Anchorena Hospital and the Buenos Aires School of Medicine. Informed consent was obtained from all the patients undergoing laparoscopic cholecystectomy for symptomatic gallbladder lithiasis between June 2011 and November 2011 [12].

The dye was administered 1 h before surgery at a dose of 0.05 mg/kg, taking into consideration the time of liver excretion [9–11]. The patients were operated under general anesthesia. A 10-mm umbilical trocar was placed under direct vision with the Hassan technique. After abdominal insufflation with CO_2, three additional trocars were inserted. The abdominal cavity was illuminated under xenon light. The gallbladder was tractioned, opening Calot's triangle, at which time there was a change of light to infrared.

Visualization was assessed with an infrared excitation system (filtered Xenon Short Arc Lamp; Karl Storz, Tuttlingen, Germany) and with a filter attached to a charge-coupled device infrared-sensitive camera with 3 chips (Karl Storz). In this way, the filters block the incident reflected infrared light, capturing only the fluorescent light. The images were obtained with the AIDA Compact II System digital device (Karl Storz).

The extra hepatic biliary duct (hepatic, cystic ducts, proximal choledochus) identification was assessed with xenon light and afterwards with infrared light. To assess the accuracy of the method, the number of patients in whom the structures were visualized before the dissection was considered to be a very positive sign. After that, a conventional IOC was performed, and specificity was considered to assess if the structures initially identified as the cystic and proximal bile ducts were confirmed by IOC.

Results

A total of 65 patients were recruited for the study (55 cholelithiasis and 10 cholecystitis). There were 35 women and 30 men with an average age of 42 years (19–73). Their average BMI was 20 (16–40). Before surgery, 6 patients had cholestasis in laboratory tests. MRI was performed. The average operative time was 120 min (30–180). The average postoperative hospitalization was 2 days (1–4).

Visualization of the Common Bile Duct

We were able to identify the common bile duct with infrared light in all of the patients. In 15 patients it was necessary to dissect the fat on the biliary tract. In 35 patients we

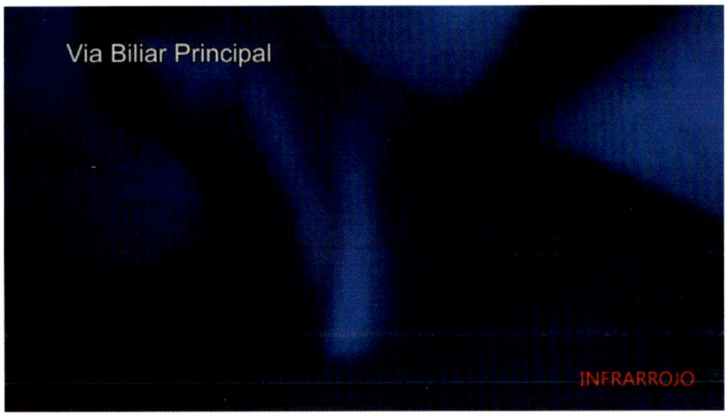

Fig. 1. Common bile duct.

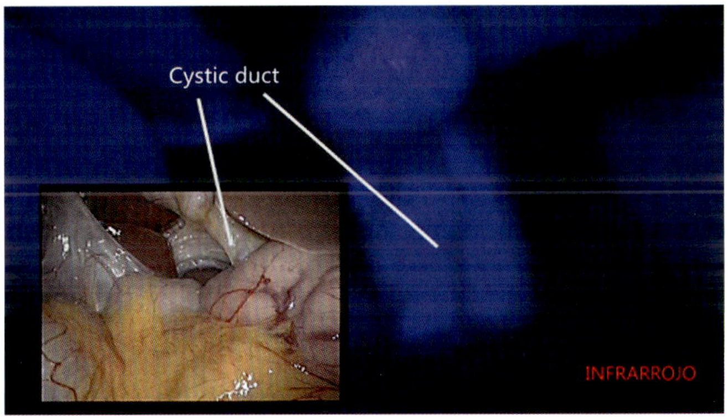

Fig. 2. Cystic duct.

found the cystic artery crossing the biliary structures (fig. 1). It was difficult to see the distal part of the choledochus in 12 patients because the dye had filled the duodenum quickly. We did not find any stones in the main structures. This was evident because the indocyanine green was surrounding the lithiasis. The structures were confirmed by the radioscopic cholangiography in all the patients. In all these cases the radioscopic images matched the fluorescent images.

In some cases, fat prevented the immediate visualization of the bile duct. The light was unable to go through the connective tissue when this was thicker than 1 cm. Nevertheless, this was not an impediment to the method since during the dissection the light worked as a guide to further locate the structures before dissection of the cystic duct and performing a cholangiography.

Cystic Duct

The visualization of the cystic duct was clear in 50 patients and required smooth dissection in 15 (fig. 2). We were able to clearly identify three different cystic arrangements: those shown in parallel, beaded and even crossing behind the main bile duct. The most important fact to point out is that in most cases before or after the dissection, it was possible to identify the choledochal cyst with fluorescence cholangiography. This fact gave us certainty during the intraoperative procedure.

Hepatic Ducts
Providing that the liver makes it possible, due to its adherence, we separated it to see the hepatic ducts. The lifting of the liver facilitated the visualization of the carrefour in 10 patients with fluorescence. Logically, intrahepatic structures were not identified.

Accessory Ducts
In 5 cases and during the dissection maneuvers and with the luminous exchange with infrared light, we were able to detect in the surgical site abnormal ducts both in the main bile duct to the liver and the gallbladder to the hepatic site which were dyed with indocyanine green and expressed as fluorescent canaliculi, which under xenon light were interpreted as lymphatic canaliculi or which were not even evident.

Bile Duct Reflux
A maneuver was performed in order to certify that the cyst was such and not just a low insertion of the hepatic duct. This consisted of applying slight pressure on the choledochus while we observed the field with infrared light. This caused a reflux of the contrast towards the gallbladder. By means of fluorescence, the luminous visualization of the contrast was generated going from the main bile duct into the bile duct, mainly in the cases when there was no lithiasis.

These preliminary data show a feasible method since it is not necessary to learn a new technique, but simply to perform a change of light. It is economical because once the luminous equipment is obtained, its implementation implies the cost of an inexpensive ampoule; it is a safe method since the drug toxicity is very low and in fact guides the surgeon to visualize anatomically the canicular structures. Further development of this method will probably generate clearer and deeper image visualization. However, although promising, it has not replaced IOC since we have not been able to detect, for example, either intrahepatic structures or the visualization of choledochal lithiasis. It is, however, complementary considering that it visualizes the structures before the section of a duct.

References

1 Rawlings A, Hodgett SE, Mathews BD, et al: Single-incision laparoscopic cholecystectomy: initial experience with critical view of safety dissection and routine intraoperative cholangiography. J Am Coll Surg 2010;211:1–7.
2 Mirizzi LP: La colangiografía durante las operaciones de las vías biliares. Comunicación en la Sociedad de Cirugía de Buenos Aires, October 5, 1932.
3 Dubois F: Cholecistectomie par coelioscopie. Presse Med 1989;18:980.
4 Cuschieri A, Shimi S: Intraoperative cholangiography during laparoscopic cholecystectomy. Routine vs selective policy. Surg Endosc 1994;8:302–305.
5 Bregante M, Iribarren C: Colangiografia intraoperatoria selectiva en colecistidis aguda. Rev Argent Cirug 2006;91:100–104.

6 Cuschieri A, Shimi S, Banting S: Intraoperative cholangiography during laparoscopic cholecystectomy. Routine versus selective policy. Surg Endosc 1994;8:302–305.
7 Flum DR, Dellinger EP: Intraoperative cholangiography and risk of common bile duct injury during cholecystectomy. JAMA 2003;289:1639–1644.
8 Z'graggen K, Wehrli H, Metzger A, et al: Complications of laparoscopic cholecystectomy in Switzerland. A prospective 3-year study of 10,174 patients. Swiss Association of Laparoscopic and Thoracoscopic Surgery. Surg Endosc 1998;12:1303–1310.
9 Ishizawa T, Bandai Y, Kokudo N: Fluorescent cholangiography using indocyanine green for laparoscopic cholecystectomy. Arch Surg 2009;144:381–382.
10 Ishizawa T, Bandai Y: Fluorescent cholangiography illuminating the biliary tree during laparoscopic cholecystectomy. Br J Surg 2010;97:1369–1377.
11 Mordon S, Devoisselle J: Indocyanine green: physiochemical factors affecting its fluorescence in vivo. Microvasc Res 1988;55:146–152.
12 Cherrick G, Stein S: Indocyanine green: observations on its physical properties plasma decay, and hepatic extraction. J Clin Invest 1960;39:592–600.

Fernando D. Dip
Oncological Surgery, Department of Surgery
Hospital de Clinicas "José de San Martín"
Av. Córdoba 2351, RA-C1120AAR Buenos Aires (Argentina)
E-Mail fernandodip@gmail.com

Kokudo N, Ishizawa T (eds): Fluorescent Imaging: Treatment of Hepatobiliary and Pancreatic Diseases.
Front Gastrointest Res. Basel, Karger, 2013, vol 31, pp 86–91 (DOI: 10.1159/000350904)

Simultaneous Near-Infrared Fluorescence Imaging of the Bile Duct and Hepatic Arterial Anatomy for Image-Guided Surgery

Eiichi Tanaka[a] · Yoshitomo Ashitate[a, b, c] · Aya Matsui[a] · Hajime Narsaki[a] · Hideyuki Wada[a] · John V. Frangioni[b, c] · Satoshi Hirano[a]

[a]Gastoroenterological Surgery II, Hokkaido University Graduate School of Medicine, Sapporo, Japan; [b]Department of Medicine, Division of Hematology/Oncology, and [c]Department of Radiology, Beth Israel Deaconess Medical Center, Boston, Mass., USA

Abstract

Two independent wavelengths of a near-infrared (NIR) fluorescent light probe are currently available in the clinical setting. These enable us to simultaneously see two different anatomies and/or functions. Many reports are available showing that NIR fluorescence imaging and merged imaging of normal light and NIR light are useful for intraoperative image guidance. Dual-channel NIR fluorescence imaging has already been reported. It has potential to provide easy-to-understand, real-time, intraoperative imaging in more detail than single-channel NIR fluorescence imaging. Indocyanine green (ICG), of which the fluorescence wavelength is about 800 nm, and methylene blue (MB), of which the fluorescence wavelength is about 700 nm, can be used for the probe of NIR fluorescence imaging with the use of an appropriate NIR camera. The FLARE (Fluorescence-Assisted Resection and Exploration) system provides simultaneous dual-channel fluorescence imaging. The results of the initial preclinical trial of dual-channel NIR imaging for a cardiac application have been published as well as the simultaneous visualization of bile ducts and hepatic arteries in the preclinical setting. Both ICG and MB eliminate into bile after intravenous injection. The nonmetabolized elimination of both ICG and MB can detect fluorescence out of the bile. Intravenous injection of ICG, MB, and their combination can visualize the hepatic arteries and bile ducts in a different phase. MB has a lower extinction coefficient than ICG, i.e. ICG is a brighter fluorescence material than MB. However, ICG has poor liver-bile duct signal contrast because ICG accumulates in the liver rapidly and persistently. Furthermore, MB can visualize the bile duct more rapidly after intravenous injection than ICG because MB shows faster elimination into bile after intravenous injection. This technology has potential to provide appropriate intraoperative image guidance that can enable us to perform surgery more safely and precisely in a clinical situation.

Recently, near-infrared (NIR) fluorescence imaging has experienced rapid expansion on a global scale [1–4]. NIR light is advantageous for intraoperative optical imaging, especially in lower backgrounds in animals or humans, than visible light. Although optical imaging is limited concerning lower tissue penetration in comparison to radiation imaging, it does have a strong advantage with regard to safety considerations for animals and humans [5].

NIR imaging also holds an advantage in visualizing anatomy and functions highly sensitively by using fluorescent probes with no irradiation. Optical imaging, especially NIR fluorescence imaging, should be one of the suitable modalities for intraoperative imaging [6], and there have been many reports of intraoperative detection of sentinel nodes [7, 8].

NIR imaging applications in the field of hepatopancreatobiliary surgery [9–11] is gradually extending in angiography, lymphatic tracking, cholangiography, and liver tumor detection. Laparoscopic cholecystectomy is one of the most commonly performed hepatobiliary surgeries. However, conversion to open cholecystectomy is sometimes necessary, typically due to unexpected anatomy, severe inflammation or adhesion, and hemorrhage [12]. We have previously described the use of intraoperative NIR fluorescence imaging to visualize the extrahepatic bile duct, as well as sites of their obstruction or injury, in real time [5, 13]. Due to possible anatomical variations of the hepatic arteries, unexpected arterial injury and hemorrhage are also serious complications of laparoscopic cholecystectomy. Additionally, if concomitant hepatic arterial injury and bile duct injury have occurred, liver necrosis, abscess, or stenosis of the bile duct may result after reconstruction. Therefore, it is better to visualize both the hepatic arteries and bile ducts at the same time to see any anatomical variation intraoperatively. Dual-channel NIR fluorescence imaging that permits the visualization of two different anatomical structures by using two different fluorescent probes can provide novel intraoperative anatomical information to improve the feasibility and safety of the surgery. An initial preclinical trial in cardiac and vascular surgery using a dual-channel NIR fluorescence imaging system has been already reported [14]. We now describe how to visualize the bile ducts and hepatic arteries simultaneously by using dual-channel NIR fluorescence imaging technology.

Near-Infrared Fluorescence Agents for Bile Duct and Hepatic Arterial Imaging

We now have two NIR fluorescence contrast agents, indocyanine green (ICG) and methylene blue (MB), which have different absorption light and fluorescent light wavelengths. MB has a 700-nm emission fluorescence wavelength with a modest extinction coefficient and about 20 μM of quenching threshold. MB is known to be eliminated quickly out of both kidneys into urine and the liver into bile in an unchanged form. The fluorescence of MB can be detected in arteries and/or veins in a vascular phase after intravenous injection and its fluorescence can be detected in urine and bile juice in a late phase. ICG has an 800-nm emission fluorescence wavelength with a twofold higher extinction coefficient and about 10 μM of quenching threshold. ICG is eliminated almost exclusively out of the kidneys into bile in an

Table 1. Optical properties of MB and ICG

Optical property	MB	ICG
Extinction coefficient, M^{-1} cm^{-1}	53,300	109,000
Absorbance maximum, nm	668	806
Emission maximum, nm	688	832
Peak CBD fluorescence, min	<5	60–90
Liver-CBD signal ratio	low	high

unchanged form (table 1). The other important optical characteristic of MB and ICG is the different signal liver/common bile duct (CBD) ratios in the early phase after intravenous injection. ICG fluorescence out of the liver is much stronger and maintained much longer than that of MB. Matsui et al. [13] reported that a 2.0-mg/kg MB intravenous injection detected CBD fluorescence over a 4 signal-background ratio and was maintained during a 2-hour observation period in a preclinical pig experiment. They also described that a 0.05-mg/kg ICG intravenous injection provided CBD fluorescence over an 8 signal-background ratio 30 min after injection and was maintained during a 6-hour observation period in a preclinical pig experiment [13].

The Combination of Near-Infrared Fluorescence Agents

It is important to take optical properties into consideration. Rapid elimination of MB from the systemic circulation and the liver has an apparent advantage for repeated injection, especially in a vascular visualization. The combination of a 0.04- to 0.05-mg/kg ICG intravenous injection 60–90 min before imaging for bile duct detection and a 0.3-mg/kg MB injection for hepatic artery detection just before taking the image is recommended under the condition that ICG and MB are the only clinically available NIR fluorescence agents, based on the preclinical data shown by Ashitate et al. [15]. The disadvantage of this combination is the adverse effect by bolus MB intravenous injection. The NIR fluorescence combination is summarized in table 2.

Detective System for Near-Infrared Fluorescence Light

The FLARE (Fluorescence-Assisted Resection and Exploration) system developed by Frangioni and colleagues provides simultaneous dual-channel fluorescence imaging. This near-future technology has been described elsewhere [14–17]. Briefly, color video (i.e. the surgical field) and two independent channels (centered at 700 and 800 nm) of NIR fluorescence emission images are obtained simultaneously and in real time, and then merged together. The NIR fluorescence images can be assigned different 'pseudocolors' from a multicolor palette and overlaid on top of the visible color video images.

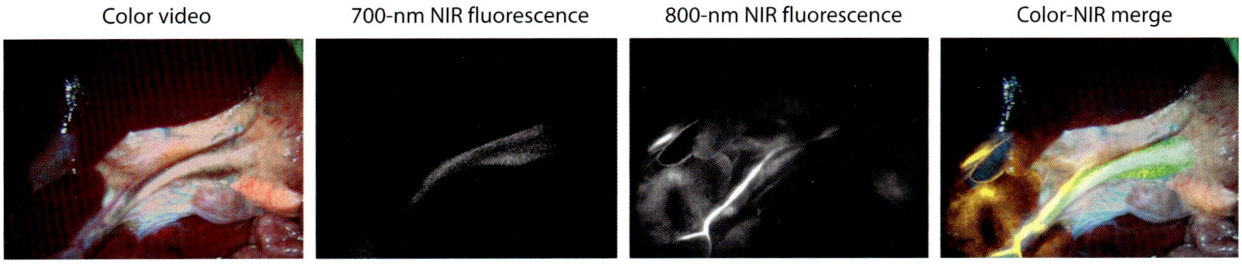

Fig. 1. Bile duct and arterial detection using a simultaneous dual-wavelength NIR fluorescence imaging system: MB 2.0-mg/kg injection 5 min before taking the image followed by ICG 0.04-mg/kg injection just before taking the image. 700-nm fluorescence pseudocolor: green; 800-nm fluorescence pseudocolor: yellow.

Table 2. The combinations of NIR fluorescence agents in bile duct and hepatic(cystic) artery visualization

Combination			Bile duct contrast agent dose	Artery contrast agent dose
ICG Injected 60–90 min before imaging	→	MB injected just before imaging	ICG 0.04 mg/kg	MB 0.3 mg/kg
MB Injected 5 min before imaging	→	ICG injected just before imaging	MB 2.0 mg/kg	ICG 0.04 mg/kg

Simultaneous Visualization of the Bile Ducts and Hepatic Arteries

A representative image of simultaneous visualization of the bile duct and cystic artery is shown in figure 1. This image can be obtained in both open and laparoscopic surgery in the preclinical setting [15]. This technology should pave a new way in the field of laparoscopic surgery in the clinical setting in the future.

Discussion

The use of two independent wavelengths of invisible NIR fluorescence light to provide simultaneous imaging of the extrahepatic bile duct and hepatic arteries during hepatopancreatobiliary surgery is a technique we will see in the near future. To maximize the likelihood of future clinical translation, two of the NIR fluorescence contrast agent combinations should be chosen from clinically available agents that are

FDA-approved for other indications in both the USA and Japan, as well as other countries.

Our recent advances in NIR technology has proven in the preclinical setting that real-time identification of the extrahepatic bile duct and hepatic arteries should be possible [5, 13]. However, differences in performance require careful selection of the appropriate combination. The goal should be an immediate clinical translation, and the second best combination should be selected based on their optical properties. The combination of MB for bile duct imaging and ICG for arterial imaging is therefore the best choice in spite of the poor signal liver-artery ratio using an ICG intravenous bolus injection. An MB bolus injection may bring harmful adverse effects in the clinical setting and nonbolus injection of MB minimizes the risk of adverse events. Furthermore, MB does not result in high liver background when imaging bile ducts. The drawback to MB followed by an ICG bolus injection is that ICG exhibits high and persistent retention in the liver, making repeated injections for visualization of the hepatic arteries increasingly difficult. To overcome this problem, Ashitate and colleagues [15, 18] introduced a 'third' contrast agent combination for simultaneous bile duct and hepatic arterial detection by using a new and improved 800-nm NIR fluorescent contrast agent for vascular visualization that exhibits no clearance through the liver with no effect of signal liver/CBD ratio. We should stress that simultaneous development of both the probe and imaging system is the key to improving this technology.

Ashitate et al. [15] also reported that simultaneous identification of the bile ducts and hepatic arteries was possible during both open and laparoscopic surgery. This technology is expected to contribute intraoperative image guidance in the setting of laparoscopic surgery. When the technology becomes optimized, the technology may also prove useful during liver resection and transplantation to guide the complex anatomy of the biliary tree, and in the future to guide cancer delineation during cancer surgery.

Conclusion

It is essential for the advance of NIR fluorescence imaging to develop both new fluorescent agents and new technology such as the NIR camera. Dual or multiwavelength detectable NIR fluorescence imaging technology can provide both more detailed structures and more detailed functional images in a surgical field during operation. Clinically available MB and ICG fluorescence can show real-time visualization of the CBD and hepatic arteries at the same time by using a dual-wavelength NIR fluorescence imaging system. We hope the application of this technology will be extended to clinical situations and cancer delineation in the future.

Acknowledgement

We thank Takeaki Ishizawa for his editorial assistance.

References

1 Tobis S, Knopf JK, Silvers CR, et al: Near infrared fluorescence imaging after intravenous indocyanine green: initial clinical experience with open partial nephrectomy for renal cortical tumors. Urology 2012;79:958–964.
2 Tobis S, Knopf JK, Silvers CR, et al: Near infrared fluorescence imaging with robotic assisted laparoscopic partial nephrectomy: initial clinical experience for renal cortical tumors. J Urol 2011;186:47–52.
3 Lee BT, Matsui A, Hutteman M, et al: Intraoperative near-infrared fluorescence imaging in perforator flap reconstruction: current research and early clinical experience. J Reconstr Microsurg 2010;26:59–65.
4 Kosaka N, Ogawa M, Choyke PL, Kobayashi H, et al: Clinical implications of near-infrared fluorescence imaging in cancer. Future Oncol 2009;5:1501–1511.
5 Tanaka E, Choi HS, Humblet V, et al: Real-time intraoperative assessment of the extrahepatic bile ducts in rats and pigs using invisible near-infrared fluorescent light. Surgery 2008;144:39–48.
6 Tanaka E, Choi HS, Fujii H, et al: Image-guided oncologic surgery using invisible light: completed preclinical development for sentinel lymph node mapping. Ann Surg Oncol 2006;13:1671–1681.
7 Crane LM, Themelis G, Arts HJ, et al: Intraoperative near-infrared fluorescence imaging for sentinel lymph node detection in vulvar cancer: first clinical results. Gynecol Oncol 2011;120:291–295.
8 van der Vorst JR, Schaafsma BF, Verbeek FP, et al: Randomized comparison of near-infrared fluorescence imaging using indocyanine green and 99(m) technetium with or without patent blue for the sentinel lymph node procedure in breast cancer patients. Ann Surg Oncol 2012;19:4104–4111.
9 Hutteman M, van der Vorst JR, Mieog JS, et al: Near-infrared fluorescence imaging in patients undergoing pancreaticoduodenectomy. Eur Surg Res 2011; 47:90–97.
10 Harada N, Ishizawa T, Muraoka, et al: Fluorescence navigation hepatectomy by visualization of localized cholestasis from bile duct tumor infiltration. J Am Coll Surg 2010;210:e2–e6.
11 Ishizawa T, Fukushima N, Shibahara, et al: Real-time identification of liver cancers by using indocyanine green fluorescent imaging. Cancer 2009;115:2491–2504.
12 Ballal M, David G, Willmott S, et al: Conversion after laparoscopic cholecystectomy in England. Surg Endosc 2009;23:2338–2344.
13 Matsui A, Tanaka E, Choi HS, et al: Real-time intraoperative near-infrared fluorescence identification of the extrahepatic bile ducts using clinically available contrast agents. Surgery 2010;148:87–95.
14 Tanaka E, Chen FY, Flaumenhaft R, et al: Real-time assessment of cardiac perfusion, coronary angiography, and acute intravascular thrombi using dual-channel near-infrared fluorescence imaging. J Thorac Cardiovasc Surg 2009;138:133–140.
15 Ashitate Y, Stockdale A, Choi HS, et al: Real-time simultaneous near-infrared fluorescence imaging of bile duct and arterial anatomy. J Surg Res 2012;176: 7–13.
16 Gioux S, Choi HS, Frangioni JV: Image-guided surgery using invisible near-infrared light: fundamentals of clinical translation. Mol Imaging 2010;9:237–255.
17 Troyan SL, Kianzad V, Gibbs-Strauss SL, et al: The FLARE intraoperative near-infrared fluorescence imaging system: a first-in-human clinical trial in breast cancer sentinel lymph node mapping. Ann Surg Oncol 2009;16:2943–2952.
18 Choi HS, Nasr K, Alyayev S, et al: Synthesis and in vivo fate of zwitterionic near-infrared fluorophores. Angew Chem Int Ed Engl 2011;50:6258–6263.

Eiichi Tanaka, MD, PhD
Gastoroenterological Surgery II
Hokkaido University Graduate School of Medicine
N15W7, Kita-ku, Sapporo, 060-8638 (Japan)
E-Mail etanaka36@gmail.com

Kokudo N, Ishizawa T (eds): Fluorescent Imaging: Treatment of Hepatobiliary and Pancreatic Diseases.
Front Gastrointest Res. Basel, Karger, 2013, vol 31, pp 92–99 (DOI: 10.1159/000348624)

Laparoscopic Fluorescence Imaging for Identification and Resection of Pancreatic and Hepatobiliary Cancer

Michael Bouvet[a] · Robert M. Hoffman[a, b]

[a]University of California San Diego, [b]AntiCancer Inc., San Diego, Calif., USA

Abstract

In surgery for pancreatic and hepatobiliary cancers, the ability to properly delineate tumor margins for complete resection is of utmost importance in achieving cure and giving the patient the best chance of prolonged survival. Correspondingly, the detection of small metastatic disease, using minimally-invasive techniques, is important for accurate tumor staging to avoid the morbidity associated with laparotomy. Selective labeling of tumors with fluorescent molecules can delineate tumor margins from normal surrounding tissue, thereby allowing improved precision of surgical resection. In this review, different methods of fluorescently labeling tumors in situ are discussed as well as the development of fluorescence laparoscopy and the potential role for fluorescence-guided laparoscopic surgery in the treatment of hepatobiliary and pancreatic cancers.

Surgery offers the only chance of cure in the treatment of hepatobiliary and pancreatic cancer. There are a multitude of factors that can significantly alter a patient's postoperative survival, such as tumor size, histological tumor grade and vessel invasion [1, 2]. However, it is lymph node status and a complete surgical resection (R0 resection) that provide the patient with the most valuable prognostic information for postoperative survival [1, 3].

As a result, targeted tumor imaging techniques have gained significant interest in recent years to enable better identification of tumors to improve diagnosis and treatment of cancer from preoperative staging modalities to optimizing the surgeon's ability to visualize tumor margins at the initial operation. Using unique characteristics of tumors for fluorescence labeling, fluorescent probes have been developed that can delineate a margin between a tumor and adjacent tissue, allowing for improved precision of surgical resection (table 1). One example is the use of fluorophore-conjugated

Table 1. Techniques for in vivo labeling of cancer cells with fluorescence

Technique	Tumor type	Fluorescence type	References
Fluorophore-conjugated antibodies	pancreas, colon	Alexa 488 or 550	[4, 5, 19, 20]
Activatable cell penetrating peptides	melanoma, sarcoma	Cy5	[8]
Telomerase-dependent adenovirus	stomach	GFP	[7, 11–13]
Oncolytic herpes simplex-1 virus	esophageal, mesothelioma	GFP	[9, 10, 21]
Targeting the folate receptor[1]	ovarian	FITC	[22]
gGlu-HMRG	ovarian	rhodamine green	[23]
5-aminolevulinic acid[1]	malignant glioma	porphyrin	[24]
ICG[1]	hepatocellular carcinoma	ICG	[14]
MB[1]	insulinomas	MB	[15]

gGlu-HMRG = γ-Glutamyl hydroxymethyl rhodamine green; ICG = indoyanine green; MB = methylene blue; GFP = green fluorescent protein. [1] These techniques are currently being used in the clinical setting.

antibodies specific for unique surface markers expressed by individual tumor types [4, 5]. Another technique is the use of replication-competent adenoviruses engineered to express the green fluorescent protein (GFP) in the presence of activated telomerase in cancer cells [6, 7, 11–13] or GFP-containing herpes virus [9, 10, 21]. Other investigators have utilized activatable probes that rely on high tumor tissue enzymatic activity [8]. In this review, we will discuss the development of fluorescence laparoscopy and fluorescence-guided laparoscopic surgery as well as its future directions and its potential use in the clinical treatment of gastrointestinal cancers.

Development of Fluorescence Imaging Prototypes and Applications

The concept of utilizing the unique replicating properties of cancer for fluorescence labeling of tumors in situ was described by Fong and colleagues [9]. A replication-competent oncolytic herpes simplex-1 virus, NV1066, was engineered to infect and subsequently lyse tumor cells selectively. In addition, this virus contained a transgene for GFP that would fluorescently label cells upon infection. In vivo infection of NV1066 resulted in localized expression of GFP to the tumor, which could be visualized endoscopically with the use of a laparoscope and appropriate fluorescence filters.

NV1066 selectively infected and replicated within esophageal cancer cells, killing the cells in vitro and in vivo.

In addition to accurately locating tumor lesions, the identification and resection of local lymph nodes is an important prognostic factor in determining recurrence and survival in patients with cancer. Fong's group further utilized NV1066 carrying GFP to infect mouse models with lymphatic metastasis of human mesothelioma cancer cells. In vitro infection resulted in all cancer cells expressing GFP. NV1066 injected into primary tumors was able to locate and infect lymph node metastases, thereby producing GFP. Subsequently, these lymph nodes were more easily visualized by fluorescence imaging. The fluorescence thoracoscopy used in this experiment [10] involved the use of an excitation filter on the light source set at 470 ± 20 nm and an emission filter on a camera processor set at 510 nm that permitted visualization of GFP.

Genetic labeling of tumors with GFP in situ has also been achieved by Kishimoto et al. [7, 11–13]. Tumors were selectively and accurately labeled with GFP using a telomerase-dependent adenovirus (OBP-401) containing the GFP gene [7] and subsequently resected under fluorescence guidance. Kishimoto et al. [11] also demonstrated that recurring cancer cells maintained GFP expression induced by OBP-401 after fluorescence-guided surgery, enabling the detection and possible resection of recurrence and future metastasis. Maintenance of label in recurrent tumors is not possible with nongenetic probes.

Antibodies have been directed against common tumor antigens to deliver fluorophores for enhanced detection of tumors during laparotomy in mouse models of pancreatic and colon cancer [4, 5]. A monoclonal antibody specific for either CA19-9 or CEA was conjugated to a green fluorophore and delivered intravenously to nude mice with orthotopic human pancreatic or colon tumors which made the tumors fluorescent. The tumors were invisible using standard brightfield imaging. The labeled tumors were resected under fluorescence guidance.

Activatable cell-penetrating peptides (ACPPs) were used as selective tumor-targeting agents. Polycationic cell-penetrating peptides (CPPs) were connected via a cleavable linker to a neutralizing polyanion whose adsorption and uptake into cells are inhibited until the linker is proteolyzed. With the upregulation of MMP-2 and MMP-9 in most solid tumors, exposure to these proteases results in cleavage and dissociation of the inhibitory peptide, allowing the CPP to bind to and enter tumor cells. Conjugating CPPs to a fluorophore then enables improved visualization of the tumor. Further conjugating dendrimers to ACPPs resulted in a higher absolute tumor fluorescence and tumor-to-background fluorescence contrast than free ACPPs [8].

Several studies have shown that near-infrared fluorescence imaging is feasible for liver-tumor imaging and segmental demarcation [14]. Due to passive accumulation of indocyanine green, superficial liver metastases can be identified with high sensitivity. A pitfall of this technique is the tissue penetration of near-infrared light, which is approximately 5 mm. This can be problematic for tumors located deeper beneath the liver capsule. Nevertheless, this technique could be of value for the detection of small superficial lesions or minimal residual tumor present after resection. Newer optical techniques are being developed to image at a depth of 1 cm or more.

Near-infrared fluorescence imaging of neuroendocrine pancreatic tumors has also been investigated in animal models. Winer et al. [15] showed the ability to clearly visualize pancreatic insulinomas using methylene blue. Intravenous administration of methylene blue permitted high-sensitivity, real-time localization of primary, multicentric and metastatic insulinomas, and enabled the distinction of tumors, the normal pancreas and other abdominal structures. Methylene blue is a phenothiazine derivative that acts as a perfusion tracer. As such, it is likely that hypervascular tumors, such as insulinomas can be visualized using methylene blue.

Development of Fluorescence Laparoscopy

With these new techniques emerging to fluorescently label tumors, fluorescence laparoscopy offers a novel method for minimally invasive cancer staging. The goal of fluorescence laparoscopy is to maximize the fluorescence signal of the tumor for easy and rapid imaging and also provide adequate background illumination to visualize surrounding tissues to allow for spatial orientation without compromising the tumor-to-background contrast. This concept not only enhances the use of fluorescence laparoscopy for diagnostic purposes, but also offers a therapeutic approach to the model.

Our group began with the development of a fluorescence laparoscope with the use of a xenon light source that would permit facile, real-time imaging and localization of pancreatic tumors labeled with GFP within the abdomen of a mouse [16]. A standard laparoscopic system was readily modified by placing a 480-nm short-pass excitation filter between the light cable and the laparoscope. A 2-mm-thick emission filter was placed between the laparoscope and camera. The use of proper filters enabled simultaneous visualization of fluorescent tumors and enhanced the diagnostic capabilities with submillimeter resolution of metastases not seen with standard laparoscopy (fig. 1) [17].

We have also applied fluorescence laparoscopy to other tumor types such as colon cancer [18]. An orthotopic mouse model of human colon cancer was established by intracecal injection of HCT-116 human colon cancer cells expressing GFP. One group of mice was used to model early disease and a second group of mice modeled late metastatic disease. For the early-disease model, 2 weeks after implantation, the mice underwent brightfield laparoscopy and fluorescence laparoscopy. The number of metastases identified within each of the 4 abdominal quadrants was recorded with both laparoscopy modalities. This process was repeated in the late metastatic disease group 4 weeks after implantation. Fluorescence laparoscopy enabled superior visualization of colon cancer metastases compared with brightfield laparoscopy in the early and late models of colon cancer. Fluorescence laparoscopy also allowed identification of micrometastases that could not be distinguished from surrounding tissue using brightfield laparoscopy.

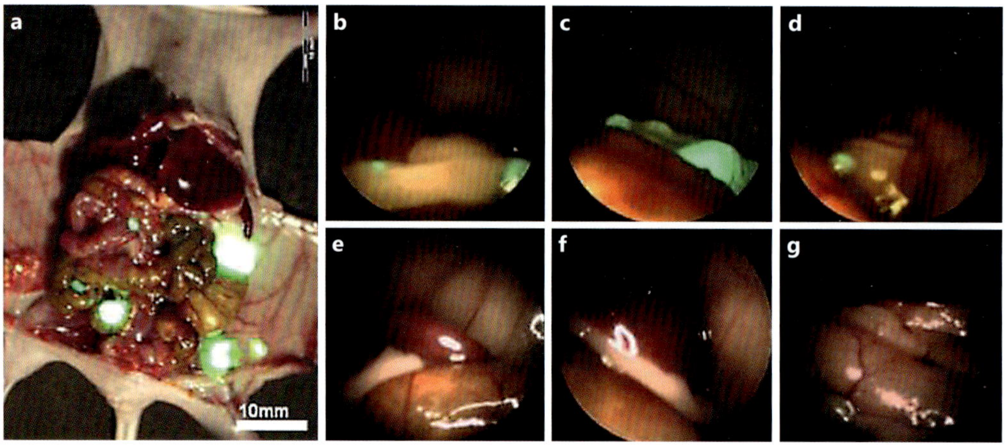

Fig. 1. Comparative identification of tumor foci under brightfield and fluorescence laparoscopy. **a** Open image from a representative mouse obtained with the OV100 small animal imaging system (Olympus, Tokyo, Japan) [25]. View of left upper quadrant in a mouse specimen under fluorescence laparoscopy (**b–d**) and brightfield laparoscopy (**e–g**). The metastatic lesion was highly visible under fluorescence laparoscopy, whereas under brightfield laparoscopy the tumor foci resembled normal tissue and were not identifiable [17].

Fluorophore-Conjugated Antibodies and Fluorescence Laparoscopy

A clinically applicable method of fluorescence laparoscopy was developed using fluorophore-conjugated antibodies directed at unique tumor antigens to label pancreatic tumors [19] that significantly enhanced the sensitivity and positive predictive value of diagnostic laparoscopy. Pancreatic tumor detection was more rapid and accurate with few false positives. However, due to the lack of intensity from the filtered xenon light, adjustments to exposure time and gain were necessary to achieve optimal imaging. Increasing the exposure time and gain resulted in significant dynamic delay that impaired surgical navigation. However, replacing the xenon light source with an LED lamp virtually eliminated the need for an excitation filter between the light cable and laparoscope (fig. 2) [20]. With only the use of a 495-nm emission filter, along with adjustments to the red, blue and green components of the LED, no further adjustments to exposure time or gain were necessary for rapid detection of a fluorescent tumor as well as visualization of the surrounding tissue for surgical navigation. The novel laparoscope produced a spectrum of light transmission that resulted in proper color balance and adequate background illumination while enhancing the fluorescence signal-to-background ratio, thereby enabling real-time visualization of fluorescence-labeled tumors and simultaneous detection of fluorescent tumors of different color [20]. The combination of labeling tumors with both Alexa 488- and Alexa 555-conjugated antibodies greatly enhanced the fluorescence signal, thereby allowing for better detection of submillimeter pancreatic tumor deposits throughout the abdomen.

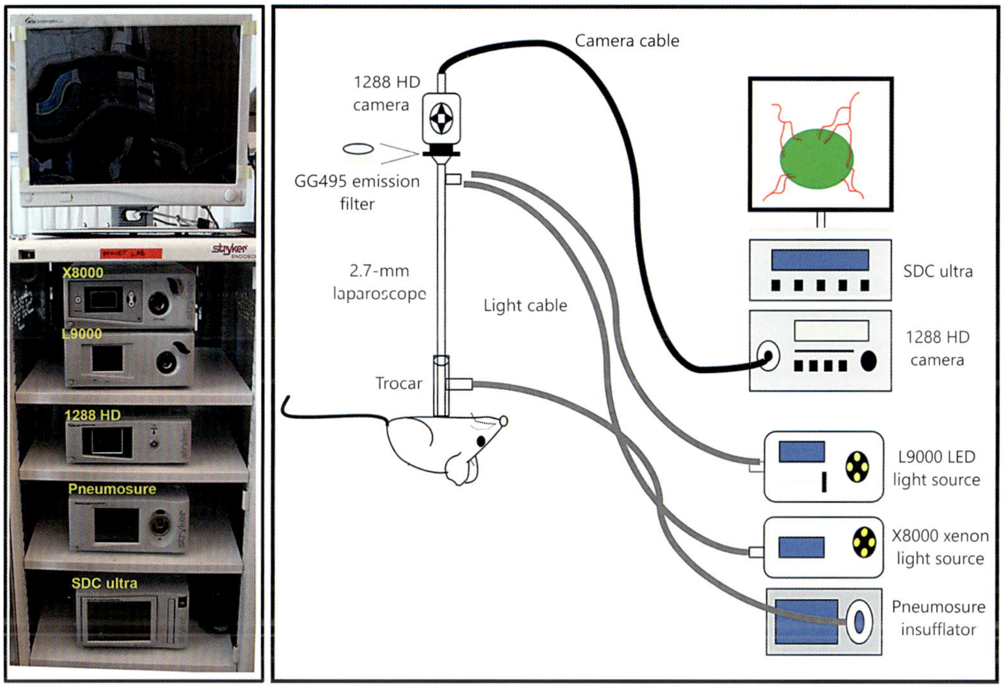

Fig. 2. Fluorescence laparoscopy setup. A standard laparoscopic tower was modified to achieve a fluorescence light mode that would permit detection of fluorescence signals while still allowing visualization of the background. The LED light source (Stryker L9000 LED lamp) was filtered through a glass emission filter (Schott GG495) that was placed between the laparoscope and the 1288 HD camera. With alterations to red, blue and green components of the light source, we were able to visualize tumors of different fluorescent wavelengths. A Stryker X8000 xenon light source was used for brightfield laparoscopy [20].

Conclusions

The ultimate goal of fluorescence laparoscopy and fluorescence-guided laparoscopic surgery is to optimize techniques of fluorescently labeling native tumors to permit better preoperative detection of metastatic tumors and to further enhance the surgeon's ability to delineate tumor margins. This will allow a more objective means of identifying and resecting all tumors at the initial operation [6].

Acknowledgements

This work was supported in part by grants from the National Cancer Institute CA142669 and CA132971 (to M.B. and AntiCancer Inc.).

References

1 Bouvet M, Gamagami RA, Gilpin EA, Romeo O, Sasson A, Easter DW, Moossa AR: Factors influencing survival after resection for periampullary neoplasms. Am J Surg 2000;180:13–17.

2 Conlon KC, Dougherty E, Klimstra DS, Coit DG, Turnbull AD, Brennan MF: The value of minimal access surgery in the staging of patients with potentially resectable peripancreatic malignancy. Ann Surg 1996;223:134–140.

3 Yeo CJ, Cameron JL, Lillemoe KD, Sitzmann JV, Hruban RH, Goodman SN, Dooley WC, Coleman J, Pitt HA: Pancreaticoduodenectomy for cancer of the head of the pancreas. 201 patients. Ann Surg 1995; 221:721–731, discussion 731–733.

4 Kaushal S, McElroy MK, Luiken GA, Talamini MA, Moossa AR, Hoffman RM, Bouvet M: Fluorophore-conjugated anti-CEA antibody for the intraoperative imaging of pancreatic and colorectal cancer. J Gastrointest Surg 2008;12:1938–1950.

5 McElroy M, Kaushal S, Luiken GA, Talamini MA, Moossa AR, Hoffman RM, Bouvet M: Imaging of primary and metastatic pancreatic cancer using a fluorophore-conjugated anti-CA19-9 antibody for surgical navigation. World J Surg 2008;32:1057–1066.

6 Bouvet M, Hoffman RM: Glowing tumors make for better detection and resection. Sci Trans Med 2011;3:110fs10.

7 Kishimoto H, Zhao M, Hayashi K, Urata Y, Tanaka N, Fujiwara T, Penman S, Hoffman RM: In vivo internal tumor illumination by telomerase-dependent adenoviral GFP for precise surgical navigation. Proc Natl Acad Sci USA 2009;106:14514–14517.

8 Nguyen QT, Olson ES, Aguilera TA, Jiang T, Scadeng M, Ellies LG, Tsien RY: Surgery with molecular fluorescence imaging using activatable cell-penetrating peptides decreases residual cancer and improves survival. Proc Natl Acad Sci USA 2010; 107:4317–4322.

9 Stiles BM, Bhargava A, Adusumilli PS, Stanziale SF, Kim TH, Rusch VW, Fong Y: The replication-competent oncolytic herpes simplex mutant virus NV1066 is effective in the treatment of esophageal cancer. Surgery 2003;134:357–364.

10 Stiles BM, Adusumilli PS, Bhargava A, Stanziale SF, Kim TH, Chan MK, Huq R, Wong R, Rusch VW, Fong Y: Minimally invasive localization of oncolytic herpes simplex viral therapy of metastatic pleural cancer. Cancer Gene Ther 2006;13: 53–64.

11 Kishimoto H, Aki R, Urata Y, Bouvet M, Momiyama M, Tanaka N, Fujiwara T, Hoffman RM: Tumor-selective, adenoviral-mediated GFP genetic labeling of human cancer in the live mouse reports future recurrence after resection. Cell Cycle 2011;10:2737–2741.

12 Kishimoto H, Kojima T, Watanabe Y, Kagawa S, Fujiwara T, Uno F, Teraishi F, Kyo S, Mizuguchi H, Hashimoto Y, Urata Y, Tanaka N, Fujiwara T: In vivo imaging of lymph node metastasis with telomerase-specific replication-selective adenovirus. Nat Med 2006;12:1213–1219.

13 Kishimoto H, Urata Y, Tanaka N, Fujiwara T, Hoffman RM: Selective metastatic tumor labeling with green fluorescent protein and killing by systemic administration of telomerase-dependent adenoviruses. Mol Cancer Ther 2009;8:3001–3008.

14 Ishizawa T, Fukushima N, Shibahara J, Masuda K, Tamura S, Aoki T, Hasegawa K, Beck Y, Fukayama M, Kokudo N: Real-time identification of liver cancers by using indocyanine green fluorescent imaging. Cancer 2009;115:2491–2504.

15 Winer JH, Choi HS, Gibbs-Strauss SL, Ashitate Y, Colson YL, Frangioni JV: Intraoperative localization of insulinoma and normal pancreas using invisible near-infrared fluorescent light. Ann Surg Oncol 2010;17:1094–1100.

16 Tran Cao HS, Kaushal S, Lee C, Snyder CS, Thompson KJ, Horgan S, Talamini MA, Hoffman RM, Bouvet M: Fluorescence laparoscopy imaging of pancreatic tumor progression in an orthotopic mouse model. Surg Endosc 2011;25:48–54.

17 Tran Cao HS, Kaushal S, Menen RS, Metildi CA, Lee C, Snyder CS, Talamini MA, Hoffman RM, Bouvet M: Submillimeter-resolution fluorescence laparoscopy of pancreatic cancer in a carcinomatosis mouse model visualizes metastases not seen with standard laparoscopy. J Laparoendosc Adv Surg Tech A 2011;21:485–489.

18 Menen RS, Kaushal S, Snyder CS, Talamini MA, Hoffman RM, Bouvet M: Detection of colon cancer metastases with fluorescence laparoscopy in orthotopic nude mouse models. Arch Surg 2012;147:876–880.

19 Tran Cao HS, Kaushal S, Metildi CA, Menen RS, Lee C, Snyder CS, Messer K, Pu M, Luiken GA, Talamini MA, Hoffman RM, Bouvet M: Tumor-specific fluorescence antibody imaging enables accurate staging laparoscopy in an orthotopic model of pancreatic cancer. Hepatogastroenterology 2012;59:1994–1999.

20 Metildi CA, Kaushal S, Lee C, Hardamon CR, Snyder CS, Luiken GA, Talamini MA, Hoffman RM, Bouvet M: An LED light source and novel fluorophore combinations improve fluorescence laparoscopic detection of metastatic pancreatic cancer in orthotopic mouse models. J Am Coll Surg 2012;214:997–1007. e2.

21 Adusumilli PS, Eisenberg DP, Stiles BM, Chung S, Chan MK, Rusch VW, Fong Y: Intraoperative localization of lymph node metastases with a replication-competent herpes simplex virus. J Thorac Cardiovasc Surg 2006;132:1179–1188.

22 van Dam GM, Themelis G, Crane LM, Harlaar NJ, Pleijhuis RG, Kelder W, Sarantopoulos A, de Jong JS, Arts HJ, van der Zee AG, Bart J, Low PS, Ntziachristos V: Intraoperative tumor-specific fluorescence imaging in ovarian cancer by folate receptor-alpha targeting: first in-human results. Nat Med 2011;17:1315–1319.

23 Urano Y, Sakabe M, Kosaka N, Ogawa M, Mitsunaga M, Asanuma D, Kamiya M, Young MR, Nagano T, Choyke PL, Kobayashi H: Rapid cancer detection by topically spraying a gamma-glutamyltranspeptidase-activated fluorescent probe. Sci Transl Med 2011;3:110ra9.

24 Stummer W, Pichlmeier U, Meinel T, Wiestler OD, Zanella F, Reulen HJ: Fluorescence-guided surgery with 5-aminolevulinic acid for resection of malignant glioma: a randomised controlled multicentre phase III trial. Lancet Oncol 2006;7:392–401.

25 Yamauchi K, Yang M, Jiang P, Xu M, Yamamoto N, Tsuchiya H, Tomita K, Moossa AR, Bouvet M, Hoffman RM: Development of real-time subcellular dynamic multicolor imaging of cancer-cell trafficking in live mice with a variable-magnification whole-mouse imaging system. Cancer Res 2006;66:4208–4214.

Michael Bouvet, MD
Department of Surgery, Moores UCSD Cancer Center
3855 Health Science Drive #0987
La Jolla, CA 92093-0987 (USA)
E-Mail mbouvet@ucsd.edu

Kokudo N, Ishizawa T (eds): Fluorescent Imaging: Treatment of Hepatobiliary and Pancreatic Diseases.
Front Gastrointest Res. Basel, Karger, 2013, vol 31, pp 100–105 (DOI: 10.1159/000348626)

Novel Fluorescent Probes for Identification of Liver Cancer and Pancreatic Leak

Suguru Yamashita[a] · Takeaki Ishizawa[a] · Yoichi Miyata[a] · Masayo Sakabe[b] · Akio Saiura[d] · Yasuteru Urano[c, e] · Norihiro Kokudo[a]

[a]Hepato-Biliary-Pancreatic Surgery Division, Department of Surgery, Graduate School of Medicine, [b]Graduate School of Pharmaceutical Sciences, and [c]Laboratory of Chemical Biology and Molecular Imaging, Graduate School of Medicine, The University of Tokyo, [d]Department of Gastroenterological Surgery, Cancer Institute Ariake Hospital, Japanese Foundation for Cancer Research, and [e]Basic Research Program, Japan Science and Technology Agency, Tokyo, Japan

Abstract

Although fluorescence imaging using indocyanine green enables highly sensitive intraoperative visualization of liver cancer through allowing visualization of disordered biliary excretion in differentiated hepatocellular carcinoma tissues and in noncancerous liver parenchyma around metastatic liver cancers, we need compensatory imaging techniques for identification of adenocarcinoma tissues during hepatobiliary and pancreatic surgery. Among numerous novel fluorescent probes, γ-glutamyl hydroxymethyl rhodamine green may have the potential to play this role through rapid enzymatic reaction between the probe and γ-glutamyltranspeptidase, which is often overexpressed on the cell membrane of cancer cells. This kind of fluorescent probe based on enzymatic reactions may also be used to detect pancreatic leaks during digestive surgery and to predict the risk of development of postoperative symptomatic pancreatic fistula, which is absolutely essential to further enhance the safety of pancreatic surgery.

Intraoperative fluorescence imaging using preoperative intravenous injection of indocyanine green (ICG) enables identification of cancerous tissues of differentiated hepatocellular carcinoma (HCC) because they can take up ICG and retain it until the time of surgery as a result of disordered biliary excretion [1]. Other types of liver cancers, such as poorly differentiated HCC, cholangiocarcinoma and hepatic metastasis from gastrointestinal cancer, do not take up ICG, but can also be detected by ICG fluorescence imaging because of the impaired biliary excretion in the noncancerous liver tissues around the tumor. However, it would be ideal if non-HCC cancerous tissues themselves could be labeled directly with fluorescent probes other than ICG.

Among the numerous novel probes developed for in vivo fluorescence imaging, γ-glutamyl hydroxymethyl rhodamine green (gGlu-HMRG) [2, 3] may have the potential to identify adenocarcinoma tissues in the liver sensitively and rapidly through enzymatic reaction between the probe and γ-glutamyltranspeptidase (GGT), which is overexpressed on the membrane of cancer cells [4]. Since GGT is excreted into the pancreatic juice, gGlu-HMRG may be applicable for identification of pancreatic leaks during surgery and postoperative pancreatic fistula formation, which is a very critical complication.

Fluorescence Imaging of Cancerous Tissues Using γ-Glutamyl Hydroxymethyl Rhodamine Green

It has been demonstrated that GGT is overexpressed in several human malignant tissues, including cervical, gynecological and digestive cancers [5–7], to promote tumor progression, invasion and drug resistance, possibly through modulation of the intracellular redox metabolism [4]. Focusing on this fact, Urano and colleagues [2, 3] developed gGlu-HMRG with intramolecular spirocyclic caging for complete quenching, which is activated by rapid one-step cleavage of glutamate by GGT, leading to complete uncaging and dequenching of the fluorescent probe (fig. 1a). In a mouse model, they revealed that gGlu-HMRG enabled rapid and real-time identification of cancerous tissues derived from ovarian cancer [2] and colon cancer [3] (fig. 1b).

Overexpression of GGT on the cancer cell membrane can also occur in liver cancers and pancreatic cancers [3]. Thus, gGlu-HMRG may have the potential to identify metastatic liver cancer during surgery, overcoming the limitations of fluorescence imaging using ICG in allowing direct visualization of the cancerous tissues of non-HCC malignant tumors. Fluorescence imaging using gGlu-HMRG may also be useful for identification of the extent of cancer spread during surgery for bile duct cancer and pancreatic cancer, if the effect of GGT excreted in the bile and pancreatic juice on the fluorescence images can be eliminated.

Identification of Pancreatic Leak and Fistula: Background

Despite the increasing experience with pancreatic resections around the world, postoperative pancreatic fistula formation still occurs with an incidence rate of 30–50%, and remains one of the most serious complications of digestive surgeries that can lead to in-hospital death following severe infections and massive hemorrhage [8, 9]. In fact, the reported operative mortality after major pancreatic resections ranges from 1 to 8% in high-volume hospitals [10–12] and can still exceed 15% if they are performed by inexperienced surgeons [13].

One of the major factors that makes it difficult to prevent pancreatic fistula formation is that no technique has been established to visualize clear pancreatic juice

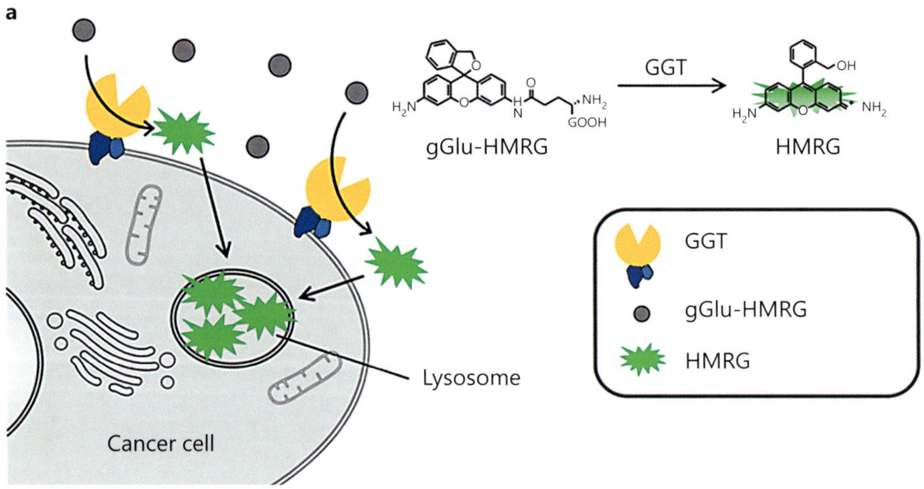

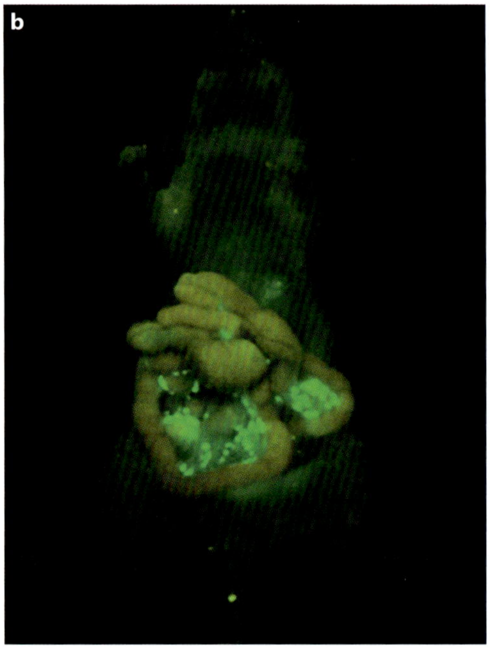

Fig. 1. a gGlu-HMRG is activated by GGT, which is often overexpressed on the cell membrane of cancer cells, and emits the fluorescence of HMRG. **b** Fluorescence imaging 10 min after injection of gGlu-HMRG into the mouse abdominal cavity identifies intraperitoneal dissemination derived from the human ovarian cancer cell line (SHIN3).

leaking from the pancreatic stump during surgery. Another problem is that no technique has been established to directly evaluate the activities of pancreatic proteases included in the drained abdominal fluids after surgery to estimate the presence or absence of pancreatic fistula formation or its severity. At present, the amylase levels in the drained fluids have been used for this purpose [12, 14, 15], probably because they can be measured easily in a hospital laboratory. However, amylase, a glycolytic enzyme, is theoretically a surrogate of the proteases that can cause tissue

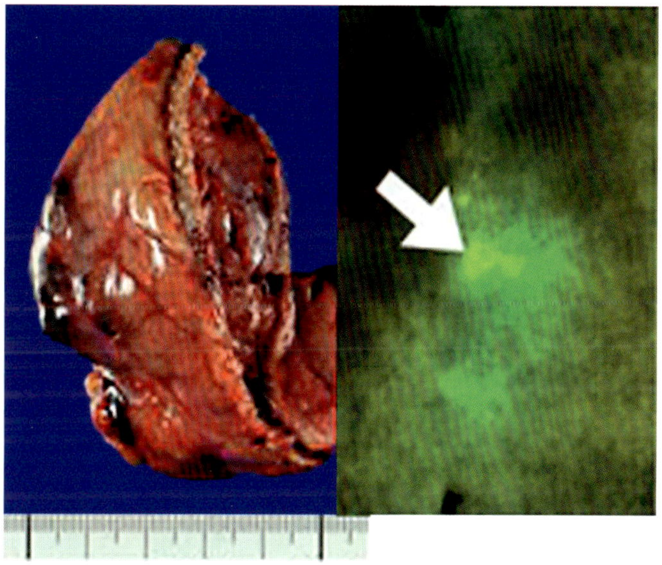

Fig. 2. Fluorescence imaging performed after applying a novel peptidase probe on a filter paper transcribing the pancreatic stump revealed a pancreatic leak spreading around the stump of the main pancreatic duct (arrow in right) that had been closed with a surgical stapler during laparoscopic distal pancreatectomy. The image on the left shows the gross appearance of the pancreatic stump in the resected specimen.

damage leading to severe postoperative complications. In fact, some authors have indicated that the amylase-based diagnostic criteria did not always reflect the severity of postoperative pancreatic fistula [16, 17]. In order to visualize pure pancreatic juice during surgery, we need a new fluorescent probe that enables visualization and evaluation of the protease activities in pancreatic juice and postoperative drain fluids.

Identification of Pancreatic Leak and Pancreatic Fistula: Technique

Since GGT is excreted in the pancreatic juice, gGlu-HMRG is a candidate for fluorescent probes that would enable accurate diagnosis of postoperative pancreatic fistula. However, fluorescence imaging of pancreatic juice targeting GGT to evaluate the severity of a pancreatic leak from the pancreatoenteric anastomosis has a limitation because GGT is secreted into enteric fluids as well as into pancreatic juice. In order to improve the specificity of fluorescence imaging of pancreatic juice, novel fluorescent probes activated only by pancreas-specific peptidases have been developed [18].

This kind of fluorescent probe based on enzymatic reactions with pancreatic peptidases may be applicable for intraoperative diagnosis of pancreatic leaks following division of the pancreas, although direct administration of novel probes into a patient's abdominal cavity has not yet been approved (pending completion of safety trials). Herein, a clinical application is demonstrated: following division of the pancreatic stump with a stapler device during laparoscopic distal pancreatectomy (fig. 2a), a novel peptidase probe was sprayed onto a filter paper transcribing the pancreatic stump of the resected specimen, and its fluorescence images were obtained using the Maestro imaging system (CRi Inc., Woburn, Mass, USA). Then, a diffuse pancreatic leak from a stapling line was visualized (fig. 2b). Since the fluorescence intensity of pancreatic leak fluid was not so high as compared with that in our previous series, no additional suture on the pancreatic stump was made and only an abdominal drainage tube was placed. Postoperatively, the amount of fluid discharged decreased shortly and the abdominal tube was removed on postoperative day 4 without any complications.

Conclusion

gGlu-HMRG is expected to delineate cancerous tissues during surgery for adenocarcinoma, complementing the ICG fluorescence imaging that enables visualization of the HCC tissues. Although fluorescence imaging has been developed mainly aiming to identify the cancerous tissues and bile ducts in the field of hepatobiliary and pancreatic surgery, real-time identification of pancreatic juice is another big challenge to be overcome in order to improve the safety of pancreatic surgery.

References

1 Ishizawa T, Fukushima N, Shibahara J, et al: Real-time identification of liver cancers by using indocyanine green fluorescent imaging. Cancer 2009;115: 2491–2504.

2 Urano Y, Sakabe M, Kosaka N, et al: Rapid cancer detection by topically spraying a γ-glutamyltranspeptidase-activated fluorescent probe. Sci Transl Med 2011;3:110–119.

3 Sakabe M, Nagano T, Asanuma D, et al: Fluorescence endoscopic detection of murine colitis-associated colon cancer by topically applied enzymatically rapid-activatable probe. Gut 2012, E-pub ahead of print.

4 Pompella A, De Tata V, Paolicchi A, Zunino F: Expression of gamma-glutamyl transferase in cancer cells and its significance in drug resistance. Biochem Pharmacol 2006;71:231–238.

5 Hanigan MH, Frierson HF, Brown JE, et al: Human ovarian tumors express gamma-glutamyl transpeptidase. Cancer Res 1994;54:286–290.

6 Yao D, Jiang D, Huang Z, et al: Abnormal expression of hepatoma specific gamma-glutamyl transferase and alteration of gamma-glutamyl transferase gene methylation status in patients with hepatocellular carcinoma. Cancer 2000;88:761–769.

7 Schäfer C, Fels C, Brucke M, et al: Gamma-glutamyl transferase expression in higher-grade astrocytic glioma. Acta Oncol 2001;40:529–535.

8 Yeo CJ, Cameron JL, Sohn TA, et al: Six hundred fifty consecutive pancreaticoduodenectomies in the 1990s: pathology, complications, and outcomes. Ann Surg 1997;226:248–257.

9 Mckay A, Mackenzie S, Sutherland FR, et al: Meta-analysis of pancreaticojejunostomy versus pancreaticogastrostomy reconstruction after pancreaticoduodenectomy. Br J Surg 2006;93:929–936.

10 Finks JF, Osborne NH, Birkmeyer JD: Trends in hospital volume and operative mortality for high-risk surgery. N Engl J Med 2011;364:2128–2137.

11 McPhee JT, Hill JS, Whalen GF, et al: Perioperative mortality for pancreatectomy: a national perspective. Ann Surg 2007;246:246–253.

12 Bassi C, Dervenis C, Butturini G, et al; International Study Group on Pancreatic Fistula Definition: Postoperative pancreatic fistula: an international study group (ISGPF) definition. Surgery 2005;138: 8–13.

13 Birkmeyer JD, Siewers AE, Finlayson EV, et al: Hospital volume and surgical mortality in the United States. N Engl J Med 2002;346:1128–1137.

14 Kawai M, Tani M, Terasawa H, et al: Early removal of prophylactic drains reduces the risk of intra-abdominal infections in patients with pancreatic head resection: prospective study for 104 consecutive patients. Ann Surg 2006;244:1–7.
15 Molinari E, Bassi C, Salvia R, et al: Amylase value in drains after pancreatic resection as predictive factor of postoperative pancreatic fistula: results of a prospective study in 137 patients. Ann Surg 2007;246: 281–287.
16 Shinchi H, Wada K, Traverso LW: The usefulness of drain data to identify a clinically relevant pancreatic anastomotic leak after pancreaticoduodenectomy? J Gastrointest Surg 2006;10:490–498.
17 Shyr YM, Su CH, Wu CW, Lui WY: Does drainage fluid amylase reflect pancreatic leakage after pancreaticoduodenectomy? World J Surg 2003;27:606–610.
18 Yamashita S, Sakabe M, Ishizawa T, et al: Visualization of the leakage of pancreatic juice using a chymotrypsin-activated fluorescent probe. Br J Surg 2013 (in press).

Norihiro Kokudo, MD, PhD
Hepato-Biliary-Pancreatic Surgery Division, Department of Surgery
Graduate School of Medicine, The University of Tokyo
7-3-1 Hongo, Bunkyo-ku, Tokyo 113-8655 (Japan)
E-Mail KOKUDO-2SU@h.u-tokyo.ac.jp

Kokudo N, Ishizawa T (eds): Fluorescent Imaging: Treatment of Hepatobiliary and Pancreatic Diseases.
Front Gastrointest Res. Basel, Karger, 2013, vol 31, pp 106–112 (DOI: 10.1159/000348627)

Novel Fluorescent Probes for Intraoperative Cholangiography

Claudio Vinegoni[a] · Cory Siegel[b] · Andrew Mlynarchik[c] · Brena Figueiredo Sena[a] · Luiz Carlos de Abreu[d] · Jose Luiz Lima Filho[e] · Jose-Luiz Figueiredo[c]

[a]Center for Systems Biology, Massachusetts General Hospital and Harvard Medical School, [b]Department of Radiology, Boston Medical Center, and [c]Division of Cardiovascular Medicine, Brigham and Women's Hospital Boston, Boston, Mass., USA; [d]Laboratory of Scientific Writing, School of Medicine of ABC, Santo Andre, [e]Laboratório de Imunopatologia Keizo Asami (LIKA), UFPE, Recife, Brazil

Abstract

Intraoperative fluorescence optical imaging of the biliary ducts has been recently shown to be an effective and economically viable imaging methodology for the prevention of biliary injury. While the exploitation of fluorescence imaging during biliary surgeries may still be relatively new, recent efforts have been made toward the development of novel near-infrared (NIR) optical imaging contrast agents with the goal to reduce unwanted intraoperative occurrences. The focus of this chapter is centered on the exploration of novel types of biliary-excreted contrast agents aimed at improving the current state of fluorescence cholangiography.

Prevention of iatrogenic injuries during biliary surgery, although relatively rare, is of utmost importance given the potential morbidity and mortality associated with such incidents [1]. During this procedure, not only is the patient at great risk for biliary ligatures, leaks or strictures, but these complications can also lead to extended hospitalizations, additional procedures and increased financial cost for healthcare institutions [2]. Such iatrogenic injuries are thought to be related, in the majority of the cases, to the misidentification of the biliary anatomy, given the inherent variability in patient anatomy and the superimposition of inflammatory changes or excess of fat around the porta hepatis [3]. Despite a controversy in its routine use, intraoperative X-ray cholangiography has been associated with a reduction in the incidence of major bile duct injury [4]. However, interpretations of its results are difficult, mainly due to the fact that intraoperative X-ray cholangiography provides information from a different point of view with respect to the operative field, which is normally subjected to continuous adjustments and manipulations during a standard intraoperative procedure. Recently, fluorescence cholangiography has been demonstrated and successfully tested in both experimental [5, 6] and laparoscopic procedures [7–14] with the use of an optical imaging system in combination with an infrared camera. While the routine use of fluorescence cholangiography depends on several factors [15], here we describe some properties of novel fluorescent contrast agents that have shown great potential to improve fluorescence cholangiography in comparison to more established existing agents.

Intraoperative fluorescence imaging is largely based on epi-illumination imaging [16]. A uniform light beam from a filtered halogen lamp or a diffused laser beam, is beam-expanded and projected onto a tissue or organ surface, while back-emitted fluorescence activity is collected by a CCD camera with an imaging lens. Superficial structures (5 mm within tissue) can be probed [16]. Tissue autofluorescence or signals from intravenously injected fluorescent contrast agents (targeted or pool) are typically exploited depending on the specific intraoperative procedure. Many complex factors need to be considered in order to achieve higher chances of success for intraoperative imaging such as: signal target-to-background ratio, CCD's quantum efficiency and dark noise, absolute concentration of injected fluorophores, choice of solute that is used with the fluorescent agent, lens magnification and numerical aperture, spectral imaging window, excitation and emission filters, and tissue optical properties. Finally, while static long exposure acquisitions offer the best images in terms of quality, the need for obtaining video frame rate information in the operative environment is heavily impacted by a poor signal-to-noise ratio.

Autofluorescence imaging modalities have been demonstrated and proven useful, although with some limitations [17]. In particular, the autofluorescent properties of bile have been investigated to determine whether autofluorescence cholangiography could be successfully performed [18]. Fluorimetry of collected bile demonstrated that excitation at 475 nm resulted in an intense emission at 480 nm, enabling real-time identification of the biliary anatomy during laparoscopic procedures [19]. Unfortunately, working at the lower part of the visible spectrum has two major consequences. First, it limits the maximum amount of penetration depth within the organs under investigation due to the strong dependence on the wavelength of tissues' absorption coefficients. Second, the autofluorescence contribution from all organs makes it very difficult to clearly identify adjacent areas. Both image interpretation and discernment of structures may then become increasingly difficult.

Administration of intravenous fluorescent agents presenting both absorption and fluorescence in the near-infrared (NIR) region of the light spectrum is therefore more preferable for in vivo fluorescent studies. In this 'optical window', targeted structures can be imaged with both increased tissue penetration and minimal detrimental autofluorescence components [20]. However, since the NIR region is nearly invisible to the naked eye, special cameras and imaging optics to capture and visualize the targeted images are necessary.

Currently, there are only two fluorescent imaging agents, emitting in the NIR wavelength range, which are approved for clinical use in the United States: methylene blue and indocyanine green (ICG). As methylene blue is predominantly eliminated through the urine, we depend on ICG, which is only excreted by the bile, to perform fluorescence cholangiography. ICG ($C_{43}H_{47}N_2O_6S_2Na$, 775 Da) is an amphiphilic NIR fluorochrome and in blood presents an absorption maximum at 805 nm, whereas its fluorescence emission peaks at 830 nm. After intravenous injection, ICG binds tightly to plasma proteins [21], becomes confined to the vascular system and is then excreted unchanged into the bile [22]. While ICG vascular imaging is already established for liver perfusion diagnostics, sentinel lymph node mapping and ophthalmic angiography, ICG biliary elimination has been successfully tested for intraoperative near-infrared fluorescence cholangiography (NIRFC) [7–14, 23].

Hutteman et al. [22] described ICG use in patients undergoing pancreaticoduodectomy. Although they were not able to distinctively visualize tumor demarcations, they obtained clear observations of the bile duct anatomy, proving the suitability of ICG as an imaging contrast agent for NIRFC. Tagaya et al. [7] also performed intralaparoscopic imaging of ICG elimination in both pigs and patients during cholecystectomy, demonstrating good visualization of the extrahepatic biliary tract.

Despite early promising results, some drawbacks make the use of ICG suboptimal for biliary laparoscopic or robotic procedures. During these interventions it is highly desirable to clearly distinguish the borders of different anatomic structures over a prolonged period of time. This capability can be obtained only when certain characteristics are present in the imaging contrast agent such as higher permeability from blood to bile, and shorter vasculature and liver excretion times. Unfortunately, ICG does not present these characteristics with the fluorescence signal appearing in the common bile duct approximately 20 min after intravenous injection [6]. Moreover, its low excretion time severely contributes to a high-diffused background component in the liver with a resulting reduced bile duct signal-to-noise ratio [15], making ICG not suitable for rapid identification of complications in an emergency scenario.

To overcome the aforementioned limitations of ICG, Holzinger et al. [18] explored the use of a fluorescent bile acid cholylglycylaminofluorescein (CGF) agent. CGF was administered to rabbits to determine its biliary recovery characteristics and to perform fluorescence cholangiography. The bile recovery rate of CGF was proven to be high, at ranges of 86–96% in doses of 10, 5 and 1 mg/kg, and bile duct fluorescence appeared 2 min after injection, enhancing the visualization of the biliary anatomy over a period of 30–60 min [18].

Tanaka et al. [24] characterized the performance of three 800-nm NIR fluorophores for real-time imaging of the extrahepatic bile ducts in both rats and pigs. Nonsulfonated (IR-786) and disulfonated (ICG) NIR fluorophores presented poor excretion efficiency and kinetics into bile [24]. Tetrasulfonated CW800-CA, how-

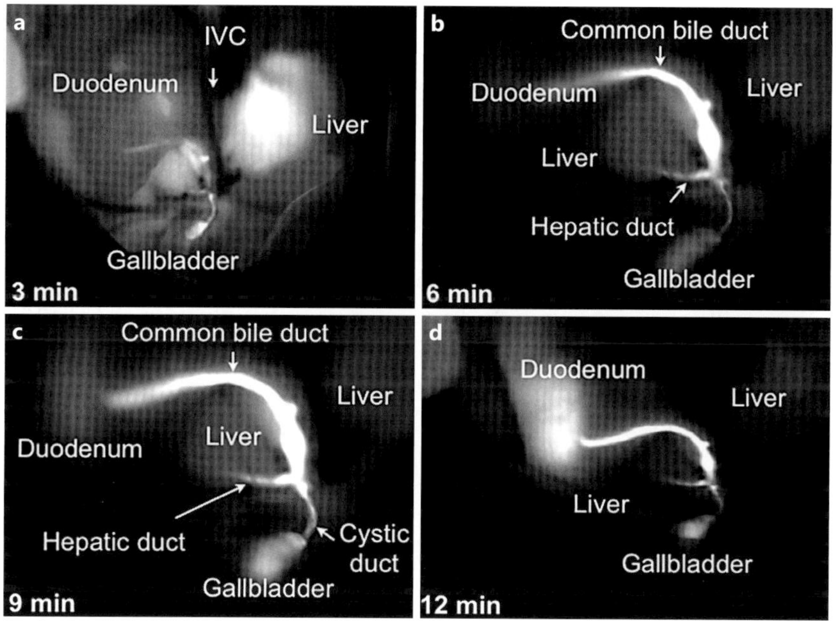

Fig. 1. NIRF images demonstrating probe accumulation in the biliary system. **a** NIRF image taken at T = 3 min after probe injection showing the beginning of probe excretion via bile ducts and comparatively low or no signal inside the inferior vena cava (IVC). **b,c** NIRF images taken at T = 6 and 9 min after probe injection, showing a high fluorescence signal coming from the common bile duct with little accumulation in the liver. **d** NIRF image at T = 12 min after probe injection, showing increased fluorescence signal in the common bile duct and duodenum with a high target-to-background ratio.

ever, provided sensitive, specific and real-time visualization of the extrahepatic bile ducts for over 30 min [24].

Figueiredo et al. [5, 15] described another contrast agent that has shown great potential for biliary imaging. VM674 (VisEn Medical, Bedford, Mass., USA) is a small molecule (molecular weight of approx. 900 g/mol) belonging to the indocyanine class of fluorophores. In aqueous media, it presents a maximum in the excitation at 672 nm and a maximum in the emission at 695 nm, with a molar extinction coefficient of 180,000/M/cm in methanol. After reconstitution in 1×PBS, VM674 was administered intravenously via tail-vein injection at a dose of 10 nmol/mouse. In contrast to 'pure' ICG, this lipophilic NIR ICG-based fluorescent agent was rapidly excreted via the biliary route, making it optimal for biliary duct imaging in mice. Using an intraoperative small animal imaging system with 649-nm excitation and 675-nm emission detection, the extrahepatic ducts were clearly visible from 3–12 min after probe injection (fig. 1) and the common bile ducts were 6–7 times brighter than the liver background fluorescence signal at 18 min (fig. 2).

More recently, Mitra et al. [25] encapsulated ICG in poly[(D, L-lactide-co-glycolide)-co-PEG] diblock (PLGA-PEG) microballoons for real-time fluorescence

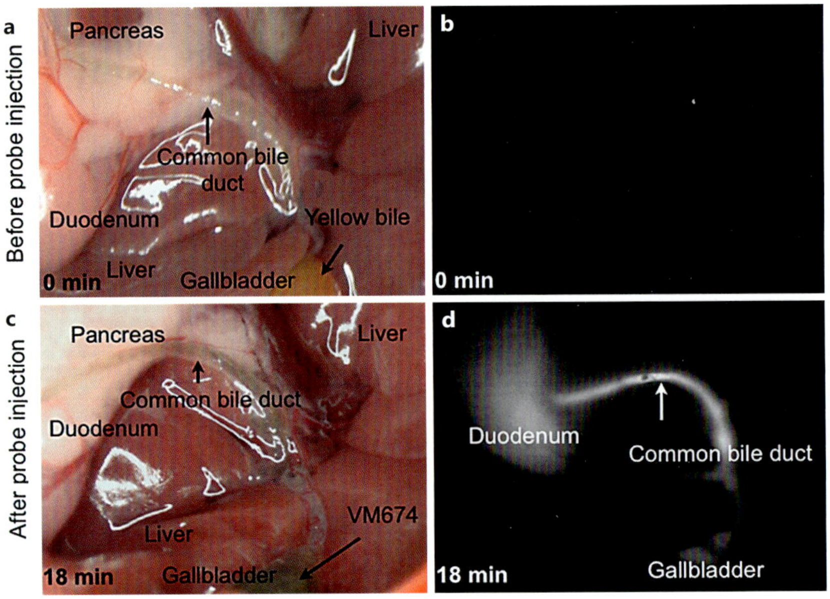

Fig. 2. NIRFC of a mouse common bile duct. **a** Color picture of the mouse liver and duodenum, showing normal yellow bile accumulated in the gallbladder and eliminated by the common bile duct. **b** NIRF imaging of the same region, before the probe VM674 is injected. **c** Color picture of the mouse liver and duodenum, 18 min after probe injection, showing the green contrast agent accumulated in the gallbladder and eliminated by the common bile duct. **d** NIRF imaging of the common bile duct and duodenum 18 min after probe injection.

and hyperspectral imaging of biliary anatomy. Using a Da Vinci surgical robot system and ex vivo models, they demonstrated that ICG-loaded microballoons show superior fluorescence characteristics and slower degradation in comparison with pure ICG [25].

Conclusion

Several investigators have recently shown the potential benefits of using fluorescent agents during biliary surgery to prevent injury and/or identify complications. Moreover, the recent developments in the design of clinically applicable NIR fluorescence (NIRF) contrast agents have improved upon prior iterations of fluorescent agents for the use in real-time fluorescence cholangiography. While previously developed techniques first relied on the autofluorescent properties of the bile in the lower wavelength spectrum, these methods suffered from high background signal, which limited their clinical utility. The introduction of NIRF agents such as ICG has improved the target-to-background ratio in recorded images, but still suffers from severe limitations mainly due to ICG's plasma protein-binding properties. Due to its prolonged blood pool phase, ICG usually stays in the vessels for an extensive amount of time (20–30 min) creating unwanted delays in the imaging process and giving rise to significant background signal from the bile's surrounding vasculature and organs.

Recently, the development of novel NIRF contrast agents with significantly improved biliary excretion time and a high target-to-background ratio represents a natural progression toward a novel class of imaging contrast agents. A functional modification by VisEn Medical (now PerkinElmer) helped shorten the time between contrast agent (VM674) injection and biliary excretion, decreased its vascular fluorescence emission contribution, and also improved the target (bile duct)-to-background (liver) fluorescence ratio in the mouse porta hepatis.

Agents with these desirable properties show great promise for the future clinical use of fluorescence cholangiography as a clinically viable and acceptable tool during biliary operations.

Acknowledgments

This project was conducted at the Center for Systems Biology at Massachusetts General Hospital and Harvard University and was funded in part by Federal funds from the Institute of Biomedical Engineering (under R01EB006432) and grants P50 CA 86355 and P01 AI 54904.

References

1 Eikermann M, Siegel R, Broeders I, Dziri C, Fingerhut A, Gutt C, Jaschinski T, Nassar A, Paganini AM, Pieper D, Targarona E, Schrewe M, Shamiyeh A, Strik M, Neugebauer EA: Prevention and treatment of bile duct injuries during laparoscopic cholecystectomy: the clinical practice guidelines of the European Association for Endoscopic Surgery (EAES). Surg Endosc 2012;26:3003–3039.

2 Törnqvist B, Strömberg C, Persson G, Nilsson M: Effect of intended intraoperative cholangiography and early detection of bile duct injury on survival after cholecystectomy: population based cohort study. BMJ 2012;345:e6457.

3 Parmeggiani D, Cimmino G, Cerbone D, Avenia N, Ruggero R, Gubitosi A, Docimo G, Mordente S, Misso C, Parmeggiani U: Biliary tract injuries during laparoscopic cholecystectomy: three case reports and literature review. G Chir 2010;31:16–19.

4 Buddingh KT, Morks AN, ten Cate Hoedemaker HO, Blaauw CB, van Dam GM, Ploeg RJ, Hofker HS, Nieuwenhuijs VB: Documenting correct assessment of biliary anatomy during laparoscopic cholecystectomy. Surg Endosc 2012;26:79–85.

5 Figueiredo JL, Siegel C, Nahrendorf M, Weissleder R: Intraoperative near-infrared fluorescent cholangiography (NIRFC) in mouse models of bile duct injury. World J Surg 2010;34:336–343.

6 Matsui A, Tanaka E, Choi HS, Winer JH, Kianzad V, Gioux S, Laurence RG, Frangioni JV: Real-time intra-operative near-infrared fluorescence identification of the extrahepatic bile ducts using clinically available contrast agents. Surgery 2010;148:87–95.

7 Tagaya N, Shimoda M, Kato M, Nakagawa A, Abe A, Iwasaki Y, Oishi H, Shirotani N, Kubota K: Intraoperative exploration of biliary anatomy using fluorescence imaging of indocyanine green in experimental and clinical cholecystectomies. J Hepatobiliary Pancreat Sci 2010;17:595–600.

8 Aoki T, Murakami M, Yasuda D, Shimizu Y, Kusano T, Matsuda K, Niiya T, Kato H, Murai N, Otsuka K, Kusano M, Kato T: Intraoperative fluorescent imaging using indocyanine green for liver mapping and cholangiography. J Hepatobiliary Pancreat Sci 2010; 17:590–594.

9 Ishizawa T, Bandai Y, Ijichi M, Kaneko J, Hasegawa K, Kokudo N: Fluorescent cholangiography illuminating the biliary tree during laparoscopic cholecystectomy. Br J Surg 2010;97:1369–1377.

10 Buddingh KT, Nieuwenhuijs VB, van Buuren L, Hulscher JB, de Jong JS, van Dam GM: Intraoperative assessment of biliary anatomy for prevention of bile duct injury: a review of current and future patient safety interventions. Surg Endosc 2011;25:2449–2461.
11 Kaibori M, Ishizaki M, Matsui K, Kwon AH: Intraoperative indocyanine green fluorescent imaging for prevention of bile leakage after hepatic resection. Surgery 2011;150:91–98.
12 Buchs NC, Hagen ME, Pugin F, Volonte F, Bucher P, Schiffer E, Morel P: Intra-operative fluorescent cholangiography using indocyanine green during robotic single site cholecystectomy. Int J Med Robot 2012;8:436–440.
13 Kaneko J, Ishizawa T, Masuda K, Kawaguchi Y, Aoki T, Sakamoto Y, Hasegawa K, Sugawara Y, Kokudo N: Indocyanine green reinjection technique for use in fluorescent angiography concomitant with cholangiography during laparoscopic cholecystectomy. Surg Laparosc Endosc Percutan Tech 2012;22:341–344.
14 Schols RM, Bouvy ND, Masclee AA, van Dam RM, Dejong CH, Stassen LP: Fluorescence cholangiography during laparoscopic cholecystectomy: a feasibility study on early biliary tract delineation. Surg Endosc 2012, E-pub ahead of print.
15 Figueiredo JL, Nahrendorf M, Vinegoni C, Weissleder R: Intraoperative near-infrared fluorescent cholangiography (NIRFC) in mouse models of bile duct injury: Reply. World J Surg 2011;35:694–695.
16 Zacharakis G, Shih H, Ripoll J, Weissleder R, Ntziachristos V: Normalized transillumination of fluorescent proteins in small animals. Mol Imaging 2006;5:153–159.
17 Tian Z, Li AD: Photoswitching-enabled novel optical imaging: innovative solutions for real-world challenges in fluorescence detections. Acc Chem Res 2013;46:269–279.
18 Holzinger F, Krahenbuhl L, Schteingart CD, Ton-Nu HT, Hofmann AF: Use of a fluorescent bile acid to enhance visualization of the biliary tract and bile leaks during laparoscopic surgery in rabbits. Surg Endosc 2001;15:209–212.
19 Stiles BM, Adusumilli PS, Bhargava A, Fong Y: Fluorescent cholangiography in a mouse model: an innovative method for improved laparoscopic identification of the biliary anatomy. Surg Endosc 2006;20:1291–1295.
20 Aswathy RG, Yoshida Y, Maekawa T, Kumar DS: Near-infrared quantum dots for deep tissue imaging. Anal Bioanal Chem 2010;397:1417–1435.
21 Vinegoni C, Botnaru I, Aikawa E, Calfon MA, Iwamoto Y, Folco EJ, Ntziachristos V, Weissleder R, Libby P, Jaffer FA: Indocyanine green enables near-infrared fluorescence imaging of lipid-rich, inflamed atherosclerotic plaques. Sci Transl Med 2011;3:84–45.
22 Tralhao JG, Hoti E, Oliveiros B, Botelho MF, Sousa FC: Study of perioperative liver function by dynamic monitoring of ICG-clearance. Hepatogastroenterology 2012;59:1179–1183.
23 Hutteman M, van der Vorst JR, Mieog JSD, Bonsing BA, Hartgrink HH, Kuppen PJK, Lowik CWGM, Frangioni JV, van de Velde CJH, Vahrmeijer AL: Near-infrared fluorescence imaging in patients undergoing pancreaticoduodenectomy. Eur Surg Res 2011;47:90–97.
24 Tanaka E, Choi HS, Humblet V, Ohnishi S, Laurence RG, Frangioni JV: Real-time intraoperative assessment of the extrahepatic bile ducts in rats and pigs using invisible near-infrared fluorescent light. Surgery 2008;144:39–48.
25 Mitra K, Melvin J, Chang S, Park K, Yilmaz A, Melvin S, Xu RX: Indocyanine-green-loaded microballoons for biliary imaging in cholecystectomy. J Biomed Opt 2012;17:116025.

Jose-Luiz Figueiredo, MD
Center for Interdisciplinary Cardiovascular Sciences (CICS)
Brigham and Women's Hospital – Kowa Pharmaceuticals
Boston, MA 02115, USA
E-Mail jlfigueiredo@partners.org

Kokudo N, Ishizawa T (eds): Fluorescent Imaging: Treatment of Hepatobiliary and Pancreatic Diseases.
Front Gastrointest Res. Basel, Karger, 2013, vol 31, pp 113–120 (DOI: 10.1159/000348628)

Endomicroscopic Examination Using Fluorescent Probes

Martin Goetz

Innere Medizin 1, Universitätsklinikum Tübigen, Tübingen, Germany

Abstract

Confocal laser endomicroscopy (CLE) has revolutionized endoscopic imaging. It permits a microscopic view of tissue during an ongoing examination for the first time. For hepatobiliary imaging, confocal probes can be introduced into the bile duct via a catheter or cholangioscope during endoscopic retrograde cholangioscopy to provide immediate microscopic evaluation of indeterminate strictures with good specificity. Such imaging within the biliary tract meets a high clinical need. Prototype rigid CLE probes have been used for confocal laparoscopy in patients with liver diseases. The use of the contrast agent indocyanine green combined with near-infrared excitation has revealed on-site parenchymal visualization of fibrosis and steatosis in patients. In animal models, CLE can be combined with a wider array of staining protocols, widening the field of scientific interrogations. CLE offers observation of fine (sub)cellular details within the normal micromilieu of a living organism over a longer period of time, and can even be combined with visualization of molecular properties of single cells. Clinical applications for liver endomicroscopy are still undergoing thorough evaluation. In translational science, the value of CLE is already well established and offers an unprecedented view into (patho)physiology.

Confocal laser endomicroscopy (CLE) is a technique providing immediate microscopic surface and subsurface visualization of tissue during an ongoing examination in vivo. Its first clinical application was described in the gastrointestinal tract in 2004 where it was used to predict the histology of colorectal lesions during endoscopy [1]. A multitude of studies evaluated inflammatory and neoplastic lesions in the upper and lower gastrointestinal tract (for review please refer to [2–4]). After the first trials showed the general feasibility of CLE and the ability of endoscopists to predict histology in vivo, follow-up trials evaluated the concept of targeting biopsies by CLE ('smart' biopsy), guiding and surveilling endoscopic interventions, and observation of pathophysiological events in the intact mucosa in vivo.

Imaging of the liver, the biliary tract and the pancreas was an early goal of in vivo microscopy, but accessibility in patients was limited. Therefore, initial studies concentrated on animal research to show the general feasibility, and only recently were followed by studies in patients.

Technique of Confocal Endomicroscopy and Staining Protocols

For gastrointestinal endoscopy, two different systems are currently registered for clinical application in humans. The first is an endoscope-based system which integrates a miniaturized confocal scanner in the tip of an otherwise conventional endoscope (Pentax) [1]. In this scanner, a single optical fiber raster scans the tissue delivering blue light (488 nm) onto the tissue and serves as an optical pinhole for emitted light (505–550 nm). This system provides a high resolution of 1024 × 1024 pixels in a field of view of 475 × 475 μm, and has a scan rate of about 1 image/s. The imaging plane depth can be user-adapted during the examination, yielding a stack of adjacent optical sections parallel to the tissue surface. A similar scanner is available in a hand-held rigid, pen-like form connected to the system via an umbilical cable for laboratory use that is compatible with use during surgery or laparoscopy in humans (Optiscan), even with different excitation and emission filters in prototypes.

The second system is a flexible probe-based system that can be passed through the working channel of most endoscopes used in patients (MKT) [5]. It consists of a fiber bundle that allows fast image acquisition at a rate of 12 frames/s, but at the price of a somewhat lower resolution. The imaging plane depth is fixed, but probes with different preset planes are available. The field of view ranges from 240 to 600 μm, depending on the probe used. The cholangioflex probe fits through a lumen of 1.2 mm in diameter. The field of view is 325 μm, the lateral resolution is 3.5 μm and the imaging plane depth is 50 μm below the tissue surface. Due to the flexible design, the probe-based CLE (pCLE) miniprobes can be advanced into the biliary or pancreatic duct, and can even be passed through a needle used for ultrasonography-guided puncture. The standard system also uses excitation in the blue range, but for laboratory applications near-infrared (NIR) wavelengths (660 nm) are available.

Endomicroscopic contrast relies on the application of fluorescent agents. Most studies of CLE in humans have utilized fluorescein so far. Fluorescein is a nontoxic agent [6] that has been used for retinal angiography in ophthalmology for decades. It is intravenously applied at 5 ml, 10%. Fluorescein has been extensively studied for flexible CLE in the upper and lower gastrointestinal tract, and also in the bile duct, liver and pancreas (see below). However, blue laser light CLE in conjunction with fluorescein showed some limitations in liver imaging outside the biliary tract [7]. Fluorescein yields good contrast of vessels and tissue architecture, but does not stain nuclei. Other contrast agents such as acriflavine, which is applied topically in gastrointestinal CLE, provide a clear visualization of nuclear structures. However, their enrichment in nuclei has raised concerns of potential mutagenetic risks, although no such adverse events have been reported with the decade-long use of acriflavine-containing disinfectants. Therefore, its intravenous use for liver imaging cannot be encouraged at present. Animal models are not limited by such safety concerns, and a wide range of topical or systemic fluorescent contrast agents has been evaluated [8].

Current Clinical Application

Endomicroscopy of the hepatobiliary system has been driven by clinical need and new developments in the field of endoscopy. Indeterminate strictures of the bile duct or early lesions in primary sclerosing cholangitis often pose a clinical dilemma. Conventional brush cytology, although having an excellent specificity, regularly shows sensitivities between 30 and 40% in clinical trials. These are higher when results are combined with other clinical imaging modalities [9], but still not comparable with other fields in endoscopy. Therefore, pCLE has been extensively studied in these patients.

In most liver diseases, histology is a mainstay in the diagnostic workup. Specimens are usually obtained by percutaneous biopsy. A sampling error for percutaneous blind biopsy in up to 30% has been reported. Therefore, macroscopic liver visualization by minilaparoscopy has supplemented histological diagnosis, increasing accuracy in randomized studies [10] and at the same time lowering complication rates [11]. However, it still relies on invasive tissue sampling and does not allow in vivo visualization of hepatocytes in their natural environment. At the same time, the introduction of natural orifice transluminal endoscopic surgery has set the stage for the advancement of endoscopes (including confocal endomicroscopes) into the abdominal cavity and onto the liver. Although most of the clinical needs have not (yet) been fully met, the following pages provide an overview of the current trials that have been conducted in the field of confocal imaging of the hepatobiliary system.

Imaging of the Biliary System

The availability of confocal miniprobes has allowed transpapillary access to the biliary (and pancreatic) tract via a duodenoscope. The confocal probe can be introduced via a catheter and guided by fluoroscopy or is placed onto the region of interest under direct visualization with cholangioscopy. Initial studies have established feasibility and shown better sensitivity of pCLE (83%) than histology (50%), establishing the presence of irregular, dilated vessels as indicative of neoplasia [12]. A follow-up study, again in 14 patients, found a somewhat lower accuracy rate for indeterminate strictures [13]. A first attempt to standardize such criteria formed the basis of the 'Miami classification' of biliary CLE [14].

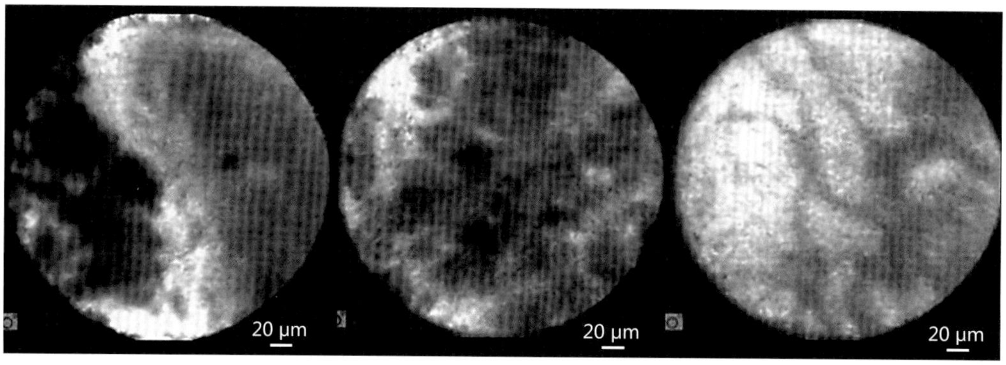

Fig. 1. Findings indicating malignancy are thick white and dark bands (left), or dark clumps or epithelial structures (middle), whereas in nonmalignant tissue, thin black structures are visible (right). Images were kindly provided by Prof. Alexander Meining, II (Medizinische Klinik, Klinikum rechts der Isar, TU München, Germany).

A recent study developed a set of pCLE criteria for indeterminate biliary and pancreatic strictures from a large data set by reviewing pCLE video sequences in a blinded fashion [15]. Findings suggestive of malignancy included thick white bands (>20 µm), thick dark bands (>40 µm), or dark clumps or epithelial structures (fig. 1). The combination of more than two criteria provided sensitivity, specificity, positive predictive value and negative predictive value of 97, 33, 80 and 80%, respectively, compared with 48, 100, 100 and 41% for standard tissue sampling methods. Although specificity was low, sensitivity (being one of the main problems of conventional diagnosis in indeterminate biliary strictures) was greatly enhanced by the use of CLE. A side-by-side comparison of pCLE findings with histopathology is difficult to obtain. Currently it is speculated that white bands correspond to blood vessels and increased neovascularization filled with fluorescein in neoplasia. Black bands may signify lymphatic vessels, and black clumps are probably epithileal structures of the neoplastic tissue. A prospective evaluation of these criteria on a background of inflammation, such as in primary sclerosing cholangitis, has yet to be performed. pCLE may be helpful in indeterminate biliary strictures to guide or complement tissue sampling since it is able to rapidly screen multiple sites with good confidence.

Confocal Laparoscopy

Rigid confocal laparoscopy is based on the FIVE1-system that has identical optical properties as endoscope-based CLE. To enable sterile instrumentation within the abdominal cavity, a rigid confocal prototype probe was developed: the scanning device in the tip was covered by a sterile stainless steel sheath and the umbilical cable connecting the probe to the laser unit was bagged with a camera sleeve [7]. The 6.3-mm blue laser light rigid probe was introduced through the right flank under minilaparoscopic control and positioned onto the liver surface in patients under conscious sedation. Serial images were generated in vivo, and some typical aspects of healthy liver and liver diseases were visualized after the injection of fluorescein. Hepatocytes, bile ducts, sinusoids and collagen fibers, as well as steatosis and pericellular fibrosis, were seen and correlated with histopathology from targeted biopsies. In addition, other organs such as the gallbladder, omentum and stomach were accessible by rigid intra-abdominal endomicroscopy [7]. However, the images could clearly not compete with conventional histopathology, other than in gastrointestinal mucosal imaging during endoscopy. This may be partially due to the thick liver capsule that did not allow sufficient penetration of the blue laser light to the liver parenchyma, or to the parenchymal (rather than layered) microarchitecture of the liver.

Therefore, in a follow-up study of 22 patients, a 780-nm NIR laser light source was used that allowed deeper imaging to 350 μm [16] (fig. 2). Since fluorescein does not show an excitation and emission spectrum in the NIR range, indocyanine green (ICG) was used for contrast. ICG has long been used in liver function tests [17]. It rapidly binds to plasma proteins and is cleared by hepatic parenchymal cells without metabolization. The accuracy of ICG-augmented confocal minilaparoscopy to predict the presence of steatosis and fibrosis was 81 and 90%, respectively. In this study, images resembling histopathological slides (including negative visualization of hepatocyte nuclei) were retrieved for the first time. However, ICG only visualized parenchymal cells and their anomalies, not inflammatory cells or biliary epithelium. Together, these studies demonstrated that liver imaging in patients was possible with confocal endomicroscopy, and showed that deep tissue imaging with NIR light helped to penetrate the liver capsule in vivo. However, other than in flexible endoscopy, liver parenchymal visualization in patients does not yet satisfy all imaging needs to compete with conventional histopathology; thus, further studies are needed.

Field of Early Exploration

Natural orifice transluminal endoscopic surgery may offer another access to endomicroscopy of the liver. pCLE was performed for in vivo microscopy of the liver and other intra-abdominal organs [18], and eCLE has also been used for intra-abdominal endoscopy of the liver [19]. The pancreatic duct has been subject to evaluation with pCLE. Surprisingly, the criteria used for differentiation of indeterminate strictures within the bile duct also seem to be applicable to pancreatic strictures as well [15]. However, further studies with a higher number of patients need to be evaluated. Endoscopic ultrasound of the pancreas has been combined with advancement of a small

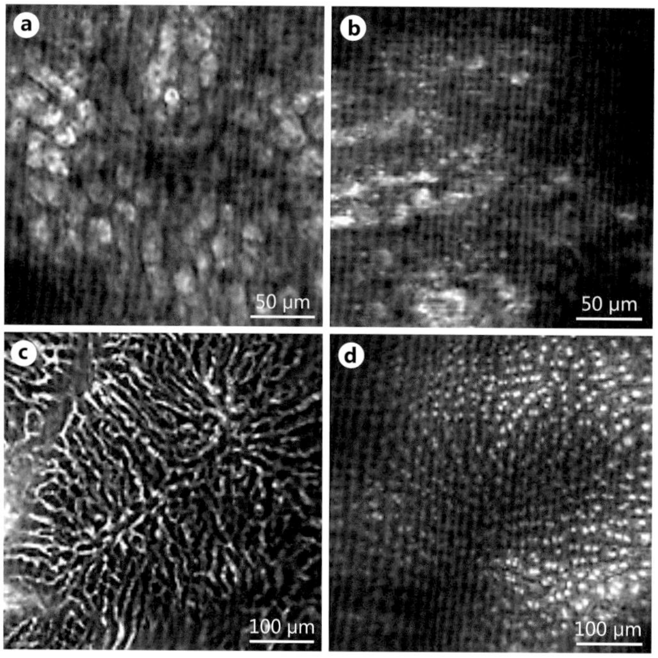

Fig. 2. a In a healthy liver in patients, the regular liver cell plates are clearly visible with NIR excitation briefly after injection of ICG, and oriented towards the central vein. The cytoplasm is bright while the nuclei are visible as unstained (black) spots inside the hepatocytes. **b** In severe microvesicular hepatic steatosis, the liver architecture is disturbed, and multiple bright spots (fatty inclusions) are visible in the hepatocytes. **c** In mice, imaging with blue laser offers different contrast agent alternatives: FITC-labeled dextrans are retained within the blood plasma and yield images of the sinusoids. **d** In contrast, injection of acriflavine stains nuclei, and to a lesser extent, cytoplasm, but not the blood plasma. Images were captured with rigid hand-held systems (prototypes: **a**, **b**; FIVE1: **c**, **d**).

probe for CLE through an endoscopic ultrasound puncture needle [20]. Such a 'seeing needle' may be especially helpful for tissue sampling in focal lesions as a guide towards the target, but has yet to be evaluated for liver lesions.

Perspectives

CLE not only tries to anticipate histopathology for in vivo diagnosis and immediate therapy, but also allows a completely new view of cells in their natural environment that is virtually free of artifacts. In murine liver imaging, this has allowed visualization of temporospatial aspects of hepatocyte apoptosis, such as identification of initial swelling (rather than shrinkage) of hepatocytes after stimulation of the extrinsic pathway of apoptosis [21]. Such aspects are difficult to capture or evaluate ex vivo or in cell culture. In addition, imaging in animal models offers a wider range of fluorescent probes that allow staining of nuclei, vessels, blood flow and other microarchitectural details (fig. 2), and permits imaging of cellular events over a longer period of time. Monitoring of extravasation of fluorescent dyes with CLE has also allowed functional visualization of inflammatory aspects of hepatitis and cholangitis [22], as well as small metastases consisting of only few cells [8]. Such detection of single-cell metastasis or foci of malignant cells within the liver parenchyma could be a promising tool to screen resection margins during liver surgery during the ongoing operation. The use of labeled antibodies as fluorescent probes for CLE has allowed identification of epidermal growth factor receptor-positive liver metastases in human-murine xenograft models by their molecular fingerprint [23]. This can be used for diagnosis of liver metastases as well as to predict response to therapy based on the visualization of the binding patterns of targeted agents.

In summary, CLE is a novel technique that is currently undergoing thorough evaluation for liver imaging. It provides a powerful tool with the potential to assist in the diagnosis of indeterminate biliary strictures in patients. Novel miniaturized probes can even be advanced through an endoscopic ultrasound-guided needle to immediately guide biopsy. In laparoscopy, prototype rigid probes have been used for imaging of liver parenchyma during minilaparoscopy. Animal models demonstrate the wide options for morphological and functional in vivo liver microscopy, and molecular imaging may open new horizons for basic and clinical science.

References

1 Kiesslich R, Burg J, Vieth M, Gnaendiger J, Enders M, Delaney P, Polglase A, McLaren W, Janell D, Thomas S, Nafe B, Galle PR, Neurath MF: Confocal laser endoscopy for diagnosing intraepithelial neoplasias and colorectal cancer in vivo. Gastroenterology 2004;127:706–713.

2 Goetz M, Watson A, Kiesslich R: Confocal laser endomicroscopy in gastrointestinal diseases. J Biophotonics 2011;4:498–508.

3 Kiesslich R, Goetz M, Neurath MF: Confocal laser endomicroscopy for gastrointestinal diseases. Gastrointest Endosc Clin N Am 2008;18:451–466, viii.

4 De Palma GD, Wallace MB, Giovannini M: Confocal laser endomicroscopy. Gastroenterol Res Pract 2012; 2012:216209.

5 Wallace MB, Fockens P: Probe-based confocal laser endomicroscopy. Gastroenterology 2009;136:1509–1513.

6 Wallace MB, Meining A, Canto MI, Fockens P, Miehlke S, Roesch T, Lightdale CJ, Pohl H, Carr-Locke D, Lohr M, Coron E, Filoche B, Giovannini M, Moreau J, Schmidt C, Kiesslich R: The safety of intravenous fluorescein for confocal laser endomicroscopy in the gastrointestinal tract. Aliment Pharmacol Ther 2010;31:548–552.

7 Goetz M, Kiesslich R, Dienes HP, Drebber U, Murr E, Hoffman A, Kanzler S, Galle PR, Delaney P, Neurath MF: In vivo confocal laser endomicroscopy of the human liver: a novel method for assessing liver microarchitecture in real time. Endoscopy 2008;40: 554–562.

8 Goetz M, Fottner C, Schirrmacher E, Delaney P, Gregor S, Schneider C, Strand D, Kanzler S, Memadathil B, Weyand E, Holtmann M, Schirrmacher R, Weber MM, Anlauf M, Kloppel G, Vieth M, Galle PR, Bartenstein P, Neurath MF, Kiesslich R: In-vivo confocal real-time mini-microscopy in animal models of human inflammatory and neoplastic diseases. Endoscopy 2007;39:350–356.

9 Rosch T, Hofrichter K, Frimberger E, Meining A, Born P, Weigert N, Allescher HD, Classen M, Barbur M, Schenck U, Werner M: ERCP or EUS for tissue diagnosis of biliary strictures? A prospective comparative study. Gastrointest Endosc 2004;60:390–396.

10 Denzer U, Arnoldy A, Kanzler S, Galle PR, Dienes HP, Lohse AW: Prospective randomized comparison of minilaparoscopy and percutaneous liver biopsy: diagnosis of cirrhosis and complications. J Clin Gastroenterol 2007;41:103–110.

11 Hoffman A, Rahman F, Prengel S, Schuchmann M, Gotz M, Moehler M, Galle PR, Li Z, Kalloo AN, Kiesslich R: Mini-laparoscopy in the endoscopy unit: safety and outcomes in over one thousand patients. World J Gastrointest Endosc 2011;3:6–10.
12 Meining A, Frimberger E, Becker V, Von Delius S, Von Weyhern CH, Schmid RM, Prinz C: Detection of cholangiocarcinoma in vivo using miniprobe-based confocal fluorescence microscopy. Clin Gastroenterol Hepatol 2008;6:1057–1060.
13 Loeser CS, Robert ME, Mennone A, Nathanson MH, Jamidar P: Confocal endomicroscopic examination of malignant biliary strictures and histologic correlation with lymphatics. J Clin Gastroenterol 2011;45: 246–252.
14 Wallace M, Lauwers GY, Chen Y, Dekker E, Fockens P, Sharma P, Meining A: Miami classification for probe-based confocal laser endomicroscopy. Endoscopy 2011;43:882–891.
15 Meining A, Shah RJ, Slivka A, Pleskow D, Chuttani R, Stevens PD, Becker V, Chen YK: Classification of probe-based confocal laser endomicroscopy findings in pancreaticobiliary strictures. Endoscopy 2012;44:251–257.
16 Goetz M, Deris I, Vieth M, Murr E, Hoffman A, Delaney P, Galle PR, Neurath MF, Kiesslich R: Near-infrared confocal imaging during mini-laparoscopy: a novel rigid endomicroscope with increased imaging plane depth. J Hepatol 2010;53:84–90.
17 Ishizawa T, Tamura S, Masuda K, Aoki T, Hasegawa K, Imamura H, Beck Y, Kokudo N: Intraoperative fluorescent cholangiography using indocyanine green: a biliary road map for safe surgery. J Am Coll Surg 2009;208:e1–e4.
18 von Delius S, Feussner H, Wilhelm D, Karagianni A, Henke J, Schmid RM, Meining A: Transgastric in vivo histology in the peritoneal cavity using miniprobe-based confocal fluorescence microscopy in an acute porcine model. Endoscopy 2007;39:407–411.
19 Kantsevoy SV, Kiesslich R, Dray X, Magno P, Giday SA, Jagannath SB, Buscaglia JM, Goetz M, Dunbar KB, Assumpcao LR, Canto MI: Translumenal intraperitoneal confocal laser endomicroscopy: a pilot study in a porcine model. Gastrointestinal Endoscopy 2008;67:AB117–AB117.
20 Konda VJ, Aslanian HR, Wallace MB, Siddiqui UD, Hart J, Waxman I: First assessment of needle-based confocal laser endomicroscopy during EUS-FNA procedures of the pancreas (with videos). Gastrointest Endosc 2011;74:1049–1060.
21 Goetz M, Ansems JV, Galle PR, Schuchmann M, Kiesslich R: In vivo real-time imaging of the liver with confocal endomicroscopy permits visualization of the temporospatial patterns of hepatocyte apoptosis. Am J Physiol Gastrointest Liver Physiol 2011; 301:G764–G772.
22 Goetz M, Vieth M, Kanzler S, Galle PR, Delaney P, Neurath MF, Kiesslich R: In vivo confocal laser laparoscopy allows real time subsurface microscopy in animal models of liver disease. J Hepatol 2008;48: 91–97.
23 Goetz M, Ziebart A, Foersch S, Vieth M, Waldner MJ, Delaney P, Galle PR, Neurath MF, Kiesslich R: In vivo molecular imaging of colorectal cancer with confocal endomicroscopy by targeting epidermal growth factor receptor. Gastroenterology 2010;138: 435–446.

Prof. Martin Goetz, MD, PhD
Universitätsklinikum Tübingen, Innere Medizin 1
Otfried-Müller-Strasse 10
DE–72076 Tübingen (Germany)
E-Mail martin.goetz@med.uni-tuebingen.de

Author Index

Subject Index